Alive and Well

A workbook for recovering your body

by

Rita Justice, Ph.D.

FOR BLAIR
Who loved me back to life

The body's a mirror of heaven:
Its energies make angels jealous.
Our purity astounds seraphim.
Devils shiver at our nerve.

—*Rumi*

Also by Rita Justice, Ph.D.
(With co-author Blair Justice, Ph.D.)

The Abusing Family
The Broken Taboo: Sex in the Family

Permissions are listed on page 297 and are considered a continuation of this copyright page.

Although the author and publisher have made every effort to ensure the accuracy and completeness of information contained in this book, we assume no responsibility for errors, inaccuracies, omissions, or any inconsistency herein. Any slights of people, places, or organizations are unintentional. The purpose of this book is to provide information that can be useful for improving a sense of physical, mental, and emotional well-being. However, as is the case with any book, it is general information and is in no way designed to serve as or to take the place of professional advice or consultation with psychological or medical professionals regarding personal health, mentally, physically, emotionally, or spiritually.

Readers are urged to use the information in this book responsibly and appropriately. Because the actual implementation of the information is, of course, out of the author's and publisher's hands and is entirely up to the reader, the author and publisher in no way take responsibility for any specific application of the information or for the results of its application. The reader is completely responsible for the application, risks, and results produced by using the information. The author and publisher specifically disclaim responsibility for those risks and results.

If readers have any questions about their ability to be responsible and appropriate with the information presented in this book, consult an appropriate mental health professional and/or physician before attempting to apply any of the information. If readers determine they are not able to use the information responsibly, do not use it. The book may be returned to the publisher for a refund.

While all examples used in this book are taken from, and are faithful to, actual occurrences, great care has been taken to protect the identity of any individuals who have not given permission to have their identities disclosed. To this end, all identifying data have been substantially altered and many examples are mixtures of several different incidents and individuals.

FIRST EDITION

Publisher's Cataloging in Publication
(Prepared by Quality Books Inc.)

Justice, Rita.
    Alive and Well: a workbook for recovering your body / by Rita Justice. — Houston, Texas: Peak Press, 1996.
    p. cm.
    Includes bibliographical references and index.
    ISBN 0-9605376-3-5

    1. Mind and body. 2. Addicts —Treatment. 3. Mind and body therapies. 4. Massage —Therapeutic use. I. Title.
    BF161.J87 1996   150
                                        QBI95-20337

Alive and Well
A workbook for recovering your body

Acknowledgements

No one recovers alone. Whether the healing is of body, mind, or spirit, it is a process that necessitates the help of others. Writing this book has been a healing journey for me. Without the support of many beloved and wise friends, teachers, family, and clients, it never could have come into existence.

To Sarah Jane Freymann, my agent and the God-mother of this book, I owe a deep debt of gratitude. She was passionate about this work long before it was anything close to resembling a book. Her encouragement and direction helped me trust myself to become a writer. That gift will go with me wherever my life's path unrolls.

My deep appreciation goes out to all my clients who taught me about the many paths to recovery. In particular, I am grateful to the members of the "Body Therapy Group." They christened the book with its title and encouraged it through its birthing like loving and experienced midwives. Diana Tuchman Burgess and Jennifer Elkins, while they were on their way to becoming psychologists in their own right, shepherded this book through its many incarnations and graciously performed the myriad mundane tasks that go into making a book a book. Their companionship and enthusiasm on the journey were a continual inspiration. Pat Caver, William Gilbert, Millie Barnes, and Blair Justice edited this book with the meticulousness of neurosurgeons and the compassion of Mother Theresa.

From its inception, I envisioned this work as an offering.

Rosalie Ramsden's beautiful design of the book is the gift wrap for the offering. Conway Adams's artistry literally made the sun rise on the cover.

Lütfiye Jeanne Herring taught me how to meditate. That much is true, but what she really taught me was how to go about saving my soul. The meditation chapter would not be in this book were it not for her compassionate and patient teaching. To her and all my teachers, I acknowledge my gratitude.

One of the great blessings in my life is to have a family that loves me. To sister Judy; my mother, Rose Alma; my brother, Paul; and and to their spouses, Rich, Ed, Liz, and their children I give thanks for that gift, the "pearl without price." My husband, Blair; our daughters, Cynthia and Elizabeth; and my stepson, David, have traveled the recovery road both with me and separately. For all that they taught me and their love, I thank them.

It's hard to know how to thank God without running the risk of sounding overly righteous or religious. Regardless of the risk, I do give thanks to the Almighty for my recovery, my body, and this remarkable life.

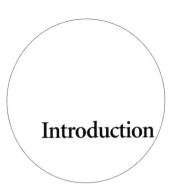

Introduction

The body has not been found. Those words, heard on the nightly news, leave us unsettled. Even if "the body" is of someone we never knew—a climber lost in an avalanche, a sailor drowned in the sea, a missing child—the incompletion is uncomfortable. The body is gone, somewhere unknown, and a mystery remains. Is the person dead or by some miracle still alive?

When your own body is lost, when the natural connection to its sensations, pleasures, and pains is missing, there is the same kind of uneasiness. You are alive but gone, present but still disconnected. Until you recover and reclaim your body, no matter how well you may be functioning, you are left with a vague dis-ease, a haunting longing for what is lost. Finding and reowning your body can bring the joy and peace of a mother who finds her lost child wandering in a nearby yard. This book is a guide to help you find your own lost body.

The first definition of "recover" in the *Oxford English Dictionary* is "to get back again into one's possession; to regain possession of something lost or taken away." To recover is to regain, acquire again, resume, or return to a condition, health or strength, or faculty of body or mind. It means to get back or find again (one who has been lost or absent). *Alive and Well* is a book that will teach you how to recover—to get back again into your possession—your body and, in doing so, to regain a sense of aliveness and well-being.

There are many reasons why the life-giving connection with the body is broken: physical or sexual abuse; shame about how your body looks; chronic or unrelenting pain caused by a diseased, deformed, or crippled body; betrayal by the body. The connection is broken if staying in the body and present to its sensations is overwhelming. Leaving the body can be a survival move. It may be the best option at the time. But choosing that option limits your aliveness and health and may no longer be necessary or possible. No matter why you left your body, you can come home to it again and in so doing find peace, safety, energy, and joy that are not possible otherwise. You can trust your body again, forgive it, enjoy it, and even love it. My purpose in writing this book is to show you how I—and hundreds of my clients—did that. It worked for us and will work for you.

I was asthmatic, allergy-ridden, anorectic, workaholic, co-dependent, and a heavy drinker. Such a biography may seem laughable, pitiable, or an exaggeration, but all those labels fairly describe my life at one point or another. Despite all those maladies, I considered myself a happy person. I had friends, traveled, did well in school, had a lover, married. I looked good:

trim, stylishly dressed, well-coiffed. I didn't see that I had any more problems than anyone else. In fact, I regarded most other people as troubled and problem-laden. I thought of myself as, if not OK, at least more OK than most everyone else. I was too well defended against emotional pain and shame to admit that much, if anything was wrong with me, with one major exception: My body ached and was ill. The allergies I had accommodated to, having had weekly allergy injections from age ten on. I half-jokingly told friends, "Just bury me with a box of Kleenex." But the asthma, bronchitis, neck and shoulder pain I couldn't ignore. They hurt and sometimes even scared me. Now I give thanks for the pain in my body. It saved my mind, my body, and possibly my soul.

The physical pain brought me back to life. My psychological armor and denial of emotional pain and addictions were so solid that only the suffering in my body could put me on the path to health. My body, not my mind or my willpower, placed me literally in the hands of a healer. Pain is a very valuable asset, especially physical pain. It insists upon our attention. Sometimes it is the only thing we have to work with that is concrete and directly knowable. Pain is the teacher indicating something is wrong, giving us a place to start repairing and recovering. Pain can be the messenger telling us exactly what's wrong.

It is possible to be so disconnected from the body and emotions that there is no awareness of pain. While there are times when dissociation is valuable and even lifesaving (see Chapter 2 on dissociation), to chronically live cut off from physical and emotional cues is dangerous and can cost you your life. People who ignore the warning signs of emotional stress place great strain on the body that contributes to deterioration and disease. Ignoring warning signs of illness, such as increased fatigue or chronic pain, keeps you from taking corrective action. It's unlikely you would have read this far if you are completely cut off from physical or emotional pain. The opposite is probably true—that you hurt a great deal. But if you are cut off from yourself to that extent, it doesn't matter. The exercises in this book may bring you first in touch with your pain. The relief and aliveness will follow. Just get started. Don't worry about what you are or are not feeling.

Twenty years ago, I developed bursitis in my left shoulder. Bursitis is a chronic tightening of the muscles, resulting in inflammation. It never occurred to me to ask, "How might this shoulder be connected to what is going on in my life?" I thought only in terms of physical pain. Even with a Ph.D. in psychology, I knew virtually nothing of the body-mind connection. One day a co-worker, weary of my complaining about my shoulder, suggested I see her bodyworker. He might be able to help, she thought. Having no idea what a "bodyworker" was but desperate for relief, I made an appointment. Lest you think I was or am someone who impulsively entrusts my body or psyche to just anyone called a healer, I assure you I approached this first encounter with a bodyworker with caution and trepidation. I think caution is advisable when one is seeking out any healer, be it for the mind, body, or soul. (In Chapter 3, I will give you my advice on selecting a therapist for the body or mind.) Now, after my more than two decades of having bodywork, the idea of taking off my clothes and climbing on the massage table to be touched by a man or woman I may never have met before still brings up feelings of vulnerability, as well it should, but I believe we all come to places in our lives where we have to risk entering the unknown. After using appropriate caution to learn what we can about a healer, we have to muster the courage to go forward and to have faith that our vulnerability won't be betrayed or violated. I had to have that faith and courage in seeing this first bodyworker.

This therapist began working the muscles of my shoulders. At first, there was more pain, followed by some relief in a few days. In the next session, a week later, he began to work on my ribs, applying hard pressure along the muscles and connective tissue. Suddenly, I began asthmatic wheezing, something I had not done for many, many years. Not only did I begin to wheeze and struggle for breath, I immediately saw scenes of the green hospital walls where I had been treated for pneumonia. I was stunned. How could that happen? In a subsequent session, when he worked on my hips, I remembered and could feel the sting of the gamma globulin shots given to me to try to improve my immune system. All those sensations, pictures, and feelings came surging back. I didn't understand what was happening, but those experiences were instant and irrefutable evidence for me of how intricately connected are the mind, the body, and emotions. I never again questioned the validity of bodywork or doubted the mind-body relationship. I was a true believer, and there was no going back. I believed then and still believe that by healing my body I would also heal my life.

In the ensuing years I have had experience with many different kinds of therapists of body and mind and have been blessed with wonderful teachers. What I am offering in this book is a distillation of those experiences that I think contributed to my being healthy physically and living life joyfully.

For almost a quarter of a century, I have been a psychotherapist. Hundreds of people have come to me for healing during those years. They come for many reasons. Some were beaten and brutalized as children. Others were sexually seduced or assaulted by parents or siblings. Broken hearts brought them. Crushing depression pushed them to my door. They came because of frantic anxiety and panic attacks, children failing or running out of control, sudden or expected deaths of loved ones, betraying and being betrayed, desperate loneliness, career defeats, physical pain that medical doctors couldn't explain or fix, chronic or acute illness, accidents and injuries. Hatred of their bodies;

shame about their shapes or physical features; being out of control of their eating, sexuality, or work had brought some to their knees and to the brink of despair. I learned from all of them. I came to appreciate that emotional healing is natural and will happen if we do what we need to do. But what has stood out for me above all else is the extent to which people ignore their own bodies as a source of emotional healing.

I have had clients who have had years of psychotherapy or sobriety and still do not feel physically well or comfortable in their own skins. Their behavior is under control. Their roles in their dysfunctional families of origin are clear to them. They have forgiven those who failed or betrayed them. All of that hard psychological work has been done. Yet their bodies ache. Those who go through medical tests usually find no demonstrable basis for the pain. Just as often as those who have never even considered psychotherapy, they take over-the-counter or prescription drugs for headaches, backaches, and every other physical malady. Even those who use less conventional approaches to healing—herbs, acupuncture, or diets—still are not necessarily connecting their physical suffering with their unhealed emotions.

I have come to believe that whatever happens in our bodies means something. A cold is not just the result of "being run down." A sprained ankle is not just being clumsy or careless or having bad luck. I don't see it as a coincidence that my client who was silently enraged at her husband broke out in an unexplainable vaginal and genital inflammation after she had sex with him. Her physician suggested the symptoms might have been caused by a virus. Perhaps, but I think her rage, not a virus, was the source of that particular inflammation. What happens in our bodies happens for a reason. The reason may be environmental, genetic, biological, emotional, or a combination of those factors. I am dismayed, though, how much people are unwilling to examine the emotional role in physical illness and how unaware they are that the body can greatly help in healing emotional illness.

I believe it is as essential to address in the therapy session anything wrong with the body (headaches, flu, a rheumatoid arthritic swelling) as it is to talk about a recent childhood memory, a dream from the night before, or a relapse of an addictive behavior. From my perspective, what happens in the body counts equally with any emotional, behavioral, or spiritual event. The body often reveals the emotions and holds the key to their release more directly than anything else.

Understanding how the body can be used to heal emotions is new even to people who have sought physical or psychological healing from a number of other approaches, including psychotherapy. Many of my clients have had a great deal of therapy. They have been in recovery programs for addictions, gone to treatment centers, been in psychoanalysis, attended marital therapy or family therapy, and followed various orthodox and non-traditional paths to healing. Some meditate. Most exercise. They have careers, families, and friends. They know a great deal about themselves, their pasts, and how they relate to others and themselves. In short, they are rewarding people to be around. So why are these healthy, functioning people wanting to do more? Most could get by without trying to understand the connection between illness, pain, and emotions. But they are not the kind of people who are satisfied with just getting by. Neither are you. When my clients find their emotions are limiting their physical aliveness and health, they want to learn how to enlist the body as an ally. They find this work of recovering the body a challenging adventure. I think you will, too. Learning to follow the wisdom of your body to healing can be an amazing journey.

When you learn to respect your body as a teacher, its instruction is boundless. Minute to minute, in response to every thought, feeling, or emotion, the Body Teacher is saying, "Good move. You got that right! Nope. Try something else. Don't do that again." The more we honor our body's wisdom, the more alive our bodies feel. For years I ignored the advice of my body not to drink hard liquor. For years I endured hangovers. Then one morning I woke up with a margarita hangover. The two very strong margaritas at the Mexican restaurant the night before were collecting their due. My Body Teacher literally pounded into my head the message "This is what happens, this is how you feel, when you do that!" I wondered why it took me so long to catch on. I never had another margarita.

The lessons from my Body Teacher continue, as they have all my life. Gradually I have learned to be a more respectful and cooperative student. My Teacher does impose many limitations and has many requirements. I don't drink hard liquor. One or two glasses of wine are permitted. Many foods are restricted: not much sugar, not much junk food. All these "requirements" came from lessons with my Body Teacher, not from "shoulds." As is my margarita lesson, I learned I simply feel better and enjoy life more if I follow the instructions.

Change isn't easy. We can ignore the body's warnings for years. But a time may come, as it did for me with the margaritas, when the pain of the hangover was greater than the fun of drinking them. It was that simple. Nothing holy or righteous, just simple math. The minus was bigger than the plus. For you to be able to invest the time and energy necessary to make changes in your body, you will have to have decided that feeling as you do isn't worth it, whatever "it" is. The great plus of feeling alive may be a little slower in coming than you would like, but it will come, providing you stick with your resolve that how your body feels now is not OK with you.

Even the most alive body cannot tell us everything we need to know for physical well-being, although it can tell us a great deal. There are no physical symptoms of high blood pressure most of the time. Arteries clog with plaque, and we're seldom aware of the dangerous narrowing that can result in a sudden heart attack. By the time cancer cells produce a lump that can be felt in a woman's breast, the cancer may have spread. Radiation can be damaging or even fatal to the body, without any physical sensation at the time of exposure. It is as important not to be grandiose in what you think you can know from your body as it is to be open to learning from it. Preventive medical checkups and necessary medical care are as much a part of respecting your Body Teacher as listening to its warnings. But the more you learn to listen to your body, the greater likelihood there is that you will be aware of subtle shifts in physical well-being and respond more quickly, even preventively.

As I become a better student, the lessons from my body get more subtle. I've learned to notice when I need to breathe more deeply, sit straighter, meditate, sleep more, exercise less. The requirements keep changing. I have no idea whether I am still in kindergarten (probably) or entering graduate school (probably not). It doesn't really matter. I honor my Body Teacher and plan to keep studying with it for the rest of my life. Healing the body is a lifelong process and an opportunity all of us have. You have that opportunity now.

In describing myself at the beginning of this chapter, I used the past tense because I am truly not that addicted person anymore. In no small part, I am not that person because I am not in the same body that carried me all those years. All the cells in the body, except those in the brain, change and are replaced every two years at least, some faster. In the brain, cells that are lost over time are not replaced, although new neuronal connections are continually being made. In less than one year, we replace 98 percent of every atom in our bodies. Physician and author Deepak Chopra says, "The body is a river of intelligence and energy and knowledge. It is constantly renewing itself. You can never step into the same river or the same body twice." From the time that I was that person I described, I have had at least ten bodies. I think it is an exciting metaphor and reality for how we are always having the opportunity to change. The Sufi poet Rumi expresses the possibility this way:

> *I am soul with a hundred thousand bodies*
> *Yet there's no "soul" or "body"; the two are myself.*
> *I've played a strange game, changed into another;*
> *This new myself's more beautiful and wilder.*

You are always making a new body you can live in. The kind of body you make today and in the future depends on what you put into it and how you treat it

now. By "put into it," I don't mean just what kind of food you consume, although that is important. What is equally important is what emotional pain you carry forth from the past into your future body. If you do not release the painful memories—emotional, physical, shameful, sexual—that are in your body, that past suffering will be part of your future and your future body, no matter how nutritiously you eat or how conscientiously you exercise.

How do you know if your body carries your psychological pain? Start by looking at your history. If you were physically, sexually, or emotionally abused, your body carries that history of abuse. Your body carries shame you feel about its appearance, functions, shape, size, imperfections, or limitations. Fear about how the body reacts, which I had every time an asthma attack began, is carried in the body. The more you now suffer physically, the greater the likelihood that the shame, fear, and abuse are still with you. All physical pain, illness, or injury has an emotional correlate. Emotions are either a contributor to or a consequence of physical illness, injury, and disease. Sometimes they are both. This is not to say that physical pain is not real. It is. Nor am I saying that physical suffering is caused only by how we think or feel. The health of the human body is far more complex than that. As my husband, psychologist Blair Justice, explains in his book, *Who Gets Sick:* "Our beliefs, attitudes, and basic positions toward life all shape the way we react when we face a threat or are required to make adjustments and changes. The way we react is expressed in our central nervous system (brain and spinal cord) and in a variety of hormones and other compounds in the body. These, in turn, affect target organs—heart, stomach, brain—and influence our immune system. Our reaction is determined not only by our basic beliefs and perceptions but also by our genes, the nature of the stress, our coping resources, our past experiences, and the context of the situation we are confronted with. Disease or dysfunction is the body's way of saying that we have failed to adapt, adjust, or change to meet the situation or that we have done so at the price of physical or mental disturbance."

New research is revealing that there is a real biological alteration in children's development as a result of child abuse. Psychologist Penelope Trickett, child psychiatrist Frank Putnam Jr., and their colleagues have found that some sexually abused girls matured earlier, had different hormonal reactions, and possibly develop impaired immune functions compared to girls who were not abused. The girls' bodies changed in response to the psychological and physical trauma they experienced. Their bodies carry their abusive history.

Emotional suffering is mirrored in the body. Where the body tightens, the pain is buried. Intuitively, we all know this to be so. We see someone who looks old beyond his or her years and think of that person as having had a hard life. Upon hearing of the heart attack of a hard-driving, aggressive workaholic, we may feel regret but not much surprise. The cues that a person is suffering emotionally are physically apparent if we look.

Postures, how we hold ourselves, are self-portraits of our emotional suffering. A stooped posture with slumped shoulders and caved-in chest reflects defeat. The body is bent as if to ward off blows that were delivered decades before to a small body that had no choice but to cower in the shelter of hunched shoulders. A puffed-out chest on a muscular trunk may be defiantly saying, "You can't hurt me." That armor-plated shield was hammered out of pain long ago. Abuse may be reflected in the eyes or face, in the imbalance between the top and bottom halves of the torso or between the left and right sides of the body. Each body carries its own story and can be the key to changing the story.

The recognition that chronic "GI," back pain, and other diseases are a sign of emotional problems is not new. What is new, though, at least to traditional Western medicine, is the idea that the emotional source of the physical pain can be reached through the body. Working directly with the body can facilitate healing both the disease of the body and the emotions.

Chronic or repetitive illnesses can be reflections of emotional suffering. Asthma, for example, which I had from childhood, is a complex interaction of physical and emotional responses. It is one of the illnesses that Western medicine and Eastern healing traditions have long known has an emotional component. Emotional suffering plays a role in so many other illnesses, too: allergies, headaches, gastrointestinal problems (constipation, diarrhea, vomiting, stomachaches, ulcers), heart disease, arthritis, skin diseases, infections, colds, high blood pressure, menstrual difficulties, eating disorders, and even cancer. This list is not intended to be comprehensive, nor is it an indictment of the millions who suffer from these illnesses or diseases. It is intended to invite you to think of physical self as connected to emotional or physical pain. Pain has more than a physical basis. All that happens in your body is an elaborate pattern of past and present coping responses. A man I know has hemorrhoids. They bleed when he's very sad or very afraid. He has a physical problem, no doubt about that, and there is no doubt for him that his emotions influence his hemorrhoids.

Extreme muscle tension is another indication that the body is carrying psychological pain. The bursitis, for example, as well as the chronic tightness in my shoulders and neck, had at its core unexpressed grief for my father, who died when I was not quite four. My tightened shoulders held back anguish and despair. Most chronic tension, I believe, is a holding of some ancient pain of emotional or physical suffering. If it isn't released, we may turn to addictions to try to cope with the pain. Marion Woodman, a Jungian analyst and author, sees repressed emotions as energies that "gain strength and may become the energies of an addiction." She warns, "Energy that is not allowed to transform toward creativity too often finds a destructive outlet."

The most telling sign of all that you are living in an unrecovered body is a sense of being empty or disconnected. Life gives little joy. Only addictions—sex, gambling, food, work—give some fleeting moments of being alive. Like campfire sparks, the aliveness is gone almost as soon as it is noticed. If you don't regain your body and release the pain it holds, sparks of life may be the best you can hope for. Addictions and pain of one kind or another will continue because they are the only source of fire, energy, and life available. With no connection to your body, you are like a rock being struck by a flint. Sparks of fire fly from the blow, but there is nothing to ignite. Addictive behaviors are the desperate and futile blows of the flint against the rock. Hope of starting a real fire that can thaw and warm and bring back life keeps the addictive behaviors going, but without the fuel provided by a recovered body, there is nothing to ignite. You give up one addiction or destructive habit and find that another has taken its place. A heroin addict becomes a drunk or polydrug user. A person gives up smoking and eats compulsively. Sex addicts become drama addicts without sex. Drunks get high on cigarettes and caffeine.

The body is determined to let you know when something is still wrong, no matter how many years you have been in recovery or how much psychotherapy you have had. The body knows not only that work still needs to be done but also what work. The body tells the truth. When it has something to say, it says it. Recovering the body means allowing yourself to learn from your own body what it really needs for recovery, regardless of what other program you are working.

Working a program, any program, is essential to

stopping destructive behavior. Psychotherapy may be necessary for emotional healing, but working the program of recovering your body goes hand in hand with other efforts at healing from abuse and psychological or physical suffering. For some people, the body is the first place to begin. If you suffer from chronic or recurring pain or illness, you may be one of those people whose door to healing will first be through the body. Whether you start with the body, mind, or emotions, recovering the body is crucial at some point to being fully well. I see it as a required course, not an elective. This is not, however, a course in immortality or in freedom from pain, illness, or death. No matter how well-attuned to the body you and I are, we are going to get sick sometimes and our bodies will deteriorate with age. We are all going to die. What is possible through this work is a sense of being fully present and alive in your body, regardless of its condition. You need not feel victimized by your body, no matter what has happened to it in the past or is happening right now. The body is not always going to offer aliveness or feel good because of structural or organic damage, and transcendence of the pain may be the only source of joy.

There is a place in you, regardless of the experience of your life or to your body, that remains pure and undamaged. It remains whole, unbroken, undefiled. That part cannot be corrupted and never has been. Author and poet Stephen Mitchell explains: "It is not that there is no distinction between pure and impure. But we are all born between urine and feces, and even in the most degraded among us, the innocence we once came from is still somewhere alive. Beneath all our pain and delusions and unsatisfied desires, it shines with its pristine light, as it did in the beginning."

Rediscovering and reconnecting with that pristine part is as essential as releasing the pain. This workbook will enable you both to lance the boil and to apply the healing balm. Both are necessary. As you re-experience the pain you have suffered, you must also re-experience the peace that has always been there. To be fully alive with a unity of body, mind, and soul, you must do both. Chapter 1 tells you how to use this book to help you do that.

How to Use This Book

"Living never wore one out so much
as the effort not to live."
—*Anaïs Nin*

You can use this book as both a first aid kit for emergencies and an owner's manual to consult on a daily basis. There are exercises for times of emergencies, like severe dissociation, anxiety attacks, or flashbacks of traumatic memories. Other exercises used on a daily basis will help you regain and sustain your sense of being present in an alive body. To get the most out of the book, use it both ways. It is meant to be just what the title says, a *workbook.* Use it step by step, at your own pace, over and over, until you feel you are in a body that is both *alive* and *well.*

Here is my recommendation for the "ideal program" for recovering your body. Clearly, there is no "ideal life," but this program is a basic one-size-fits-all that you can adapt, alter, and accessorize to fit your own life. This basic plan for using the book and recovering your body maximizes benefit and minimizes expenditure of time. Everyone is busy, and few people have the luxury of setting aside large blocks of time on a regular basis for any healing task. Recovering your body doesn't require you to alter your lifestyle radically. More than anything else, it is an alteration of your awareness.

Begin by thinking about your body more often. Having a copy of this book handy— in your purse, by your bed, in a briefcase, even on your desk— will help. As soon as you have finished reading the Introduction and this chapter on how to use the book, read Chapters 4 and 5, "Start Breathing" and "Get Moving." You can read the other chapters later. The most important thing is to start now getting back into your body. Breathing and moving are the most immediate ways of doing that. Do the first exercise, *Watch Your Breath,* in Chapter 4. It takes only a few minutes and will immediately help you to become more aware of how you are (or aren't) breathing. Next do the first exercise, *Shake It Up,* in Chapter 5. You'll feel lighter and looser in just the few minutes it takes. That's it for Day 1. If you're too busy to do any more reading in this book for a few days (or even weeks), keep repeating those two exercises on a daily basis if you can. When you have time to read again, do the next exercises in Chapters 4 and 5. Every day do one exercise in breathing and one in moving. Once you've learned how to breathe more freely, you don't need to set aside any extra time. Just breathe, no matter what else you're doing. The same goes for moving. As you become more conscious of your body movement or lack thereof, you automatically will start to make more adjustments.

Aim for trying one new exercise a week. Don't rush through or put a time pressure on yourself. Fit the exercises into your life. Some exercises you may need right now, particularly if you're losing yourself or dissociating a great deal. Chapter 6, "Get Grounded," has exercises that will help you settle down when you are "out of it" or "wired." The exercises in that chapter take only a few minutes and help immediately. But start with the breathing and moving exercises. They are the basics.

There are times for all of us when everything falls apart and no regimen is possible. On those days or weeks, do just one thing for your body. Do the *Shake it Up* exercise in Chapter 5. Let it be your security blanket that you grab when you need the comfort and reassurance that you and your body are still one. Don't worry if you get sidetracked in this work of recovering your body. Guilt is optional. Skip it if you can. Remember that as long as you have a body, you have the opportunity to reclaim it. The course is over only when you take in your last breath. Until then, class is still in session. It's never too late, and you can never be too far behind to make it worth the effort. So keep this book open, do your homework as faithfully as possible, and take credit for the well-deserved results you'll receive.

The exercises in this book are for the purpose of awakening your awareness of your body, helping you to reconnect with it, and facilitating the release of held-in emotions. The emotions you release at first may be painful, possibly as painful as when you first experienced them. Understandably, you may be afraid to lance the boil. Be as brave as you can be while at the same time being gentle and kind to yourself. Take your time. The exercises are arranged so that you can begin very slowly. There's no need for force or rushing. Both will be counterproductive.

While these exercises will be beneficial to you at many levels, they are not a substitute for giving your body regular exercise. Some kind of vigorous exercise three times a week should be a goal. That exercise could be yoga, jogging, fast walking, swimming, T'ai Chi, dancing, sports. What you choose depends on you. I jog and also go to yoga classes several times a week because I like the balance of the two types of movement and exercise. But you may not have the opportunity for, or interest in, doing that much exercise. It isn't necessary. For those of you who already feel overscheduled and overcommitted, it may seem like an impossible stretch to add regular exercise to your regimen. That's what I recommend, though. Just thirty minutes three times a week is enough. Paradoxically, the time you spend exercising will give you more time to spend in other ways.

The "extra" time comes from feeling more energy, being able to work more efficiently, and having to spend less time in other stress-relieving activities, like sleeping, "happy hour," or TV-watching. Time spent exercising is an investment that pays both immediate and long-term dividends.

The course of recovering your body is never short or easy. Staying sober if you are an alcoholic, staying clean if you are a drug addict, or controlling your food intake if you are a compulsive eater is not easy. Maybe it shouldn't be. We sometimes miss the value in what comes too easily. But this isn't impossibly difficult either. Recovering your body is a challenge, like climbing a mountain. It does require effort sometimes and is a great adventure the entire time.

Climbing mountains is work, but my husband, Blair, and I love to do it. One summer we climbed Long's Peak in Colorado. It is more than 14,000 feet high and famous for its legends of heroic climbers in this century and the last. Despite the arduousness, thousands of people climb to the top each summer. Not just experienced mountaineers but all kinds of folks climb it: adolescents in jogging shoes, groups of young women friends, sturdy senior citizens, middle-aged former yuppies. They all set out with a goal and commitment. Some make it as far as they had planned; others don't for a variety of reasons (wrong clothes, changes in weather, fatigue, running out of time). No matter how far anyone gets, there is only one way to do it—one step at a time. Follow the signs, stay on the trail, and put one foot in front of the other. Also rest when needed. Enjoy the vistas. Enjoy the flowers and fresh air along the way. Don't be so intent on getting to some distant peak that you miss the satisfaction of climbing over each boulder and fording the streams. Be prepared for the unexpected. Keep breathing. Keep going. That's what it takes to climb Long's Peak—and to recover your body.

Our round trip to the top of Long's Peak began and ended in the moonlight. We hiked and climbed more than fourteen hours. I felt the whole rainbow of feelings: anticipation, fear, frustration, joy, ecstasy, satisfaction, peace, sadness, bliss, fatigue. Despite the rigor of the journey, I never considered giving up. I wasn't trying to prove anything. I was just doing it. As the hours and miles passed, it became clear that the journey was a spiritual as much as a physical one and that we were heading somewhere way beyond a mountaintop. I'm sure many of the thousands of other climbers who have trodden those paths and scrambled over the boulders felt the same way.

Recovering your body can be a spiritual journey, too. It may become that even if you don't intend or want it to be. By spiritual, I mean having a connection with some transcendent Presence, something that is larger than you and contains you. As you are freed of the pain held in your body, you are very likely to experience more and more of that Presence. You don't have to try to make it happen. Just do the work, take the steps, make the climb.

I have a client who consciously chooses the hard path. She says, "I know if I choose the easy way, I will always have regrets that I didn't do the right thing. When I know what the right thing is, I make myself do it. I feel I have to if I am to have integrity." She sees herself as having no other option. Maybe none of us does. In the last accounting, if we are going to be who we are, at some point we have to do the hard thing, to face what we run from. Taking the steps to recover your body is facing the pain that will otherwise haunt you wherever you go. So be as brave as you can. Many others have climbed this mountain and reported amazing vistas. Those vistas can be summed up as "peace which passeth all understanding."

The exercises in this book are a path to reexperiencing with the body its wisdom, the pain it holds, the blocked expression of that pain and wholeness. By doing the exercises, your body, mind, and emotions come back together. The process is a gradual one and requires some patience. As one psychophysical therapist cautions, "The body is a metaphor for where you are in life. Challenging the body to change is challenging the personality." But there are immediate rewards: feeling more relaxed, experiencing less muscular tension, and having more energy. The big changes come more slowly, as they should. This work is similar to an archeological dig, with slow uncarthing of layers of buried memories and emotions and a persistent piecing together of broken shards into a whole vessel. The dig is a lifelong project. This process is illustrated by an example of a client of mine, whom I will call "Sarah."

Sarah had no memory of having been sexually abused as a child. She did have severe depression, which is what brought her to see me. When we first began the work to help her connect her body with her emotions, I instructed her in gentle breathing exercises. Just through the simple process of taking in deep breaths, she had a total-body response of fear. She would duck her head, wrap her arms around herself, clench her jaws, and shut her eyes. Instantly she contracted and shut down to protect herself. Later we began doing exercises that entailed some physical movement. She still felt fear but began to be more aware of differences in sensations, specifically the sensation of hands being all over her. So instead of her whole body's responding with contraction and fear, she could discriminate sensations that she was not aware of before.

Gradually, through exercises of breathing and moving, she began to remember fragments of images—a man's face; a white room; a cold, hard table. Eventually, as some of her buried terror, pain, and rage were released, Sarah remembered whole scenes involving her father, mother, and others. Over a period of time, she came to the inescapable understanding that she had been sexually abused and horribly mistreated. Sarah was able to recall the memory of being pulled into a closet and raped by her father when she was three. Now Sarah registers more subtle body sensations at the time they are happening. She can feel her body sensing fear, contracting, and then releasing in relief. Her awareness is much more refined. She feels what happens as it happens.

The benefits of this work are not only for people like Sarah, who have been seriously abused. No matter why you quit trusting and loving your body, you can learn to put confidence in it again. Helen lost confidence in her body when she developed an inner-ear disorder that left her with unpredictable dizziness and nausea. Tom felt betrayed by his body because it stopped growing when he was only five feet tall. Lisa's dream of being a ballerina was crushed when she was five by childhood rheumatoid arthritis. Bob cut off his finger in a woodworking class when he was sixteen. From then on, he hid his hand and the shame he felt about it any way he could. Elizabeth was terrified that her body would continue to erupt in paralyzing anxiety attacks. All of these clients of mine benefitted from the exercises in the book. They no longer fear, distrust, or hate their bodies. Emotional healing has taken place even when physical curing was not possible. For many of them and others, healing has been on both an emotional and a physical level.

Recovery of the body necessitates having a tolerance for the back-and-forth process of releasing and resisting, slowly coming back to an aliveness. You feel the pain and want to stop, but if you can stay with the pain until it lessens or releases, you will feel better and more willing to go farther the next time. Like getting through any of life's pain, it is a process that necessitates patience and courage. The unconscious allows us to remember and experience only so much at a time. To do otherwise would be overwhelming. Even without childhood abuse or body shame, remembering all the ordinary trauma of childhood at once would be too much. Every fall, every belly-buster off the high-diving board, every conked head—we would simply be overwhelmed if all those painful memories were felt at the same time. The memories have to come gradually. The process takes courage because the pain comes before the relief. Courage and faith are essential for us to be able to allow the painful memories to surface. Aliveness, better health, more energy, more joy are the prizes, but going through the pain is the price.

Each act of experiencing pain needs to be followed by some healing relief. At the end of many of the exercises is a brief imagery for applying that healing balm. Please don't skip it in the interest of time. It is the ointment of love you put on the opened wound that has just been cleaned. Accessing the undamaged purity in yourself will speed the healing and your recovery.

Expect setbacks in the process of recovering your body. Researchers say people change addictive behaviors by progressing through five stages. These stages are: Precontemplation, Contemplation, Preparation,

Action, and Maintenance. Recycling through these stages several times is typical before one gives up an addiction. Allow yourself plenty of opportunities for recycling through the stages. Precontemplation is the stage of denial. You don't see any problem with your body and have no intention of changing. If enough pressure is applied by others, you might change somewhat, but the change will last only as long as the pressure is on. That's not where you are now or you wouldn't have read this far in this book. But you might hit precontemplation again and decide that all this body-recovery stuff is hogwash. Contemplation, the next stage in the change process, is your awareness that a problem exists and your serious thought about overcoming it but without a commitment to do anything, to take action. Contemplation is a period of weighing the pros and cons of changing. If you haven't started any of the breathing or movement exercises yet, this may be where you are.

In the Preparation stage, you have made some small behavioral changes but are not yet ready to take effective action, for example, doing a breathing exercise one day but forgetting about it until a week or two later. In the Action stage, you do or change what is necessary to recover your body—following the prescriptions I outline in this chapter. We know that, action requires considerable commitment of time and energy. Maintenance is the final stage when you work to keep your body and emotions connected and to build on successes you already have achieved. This final stage lasts a lifetime. Relapse and recycling through the stages is common as you try to change, modify, or stop any addictive or destructive behavior.

What all this means is that change is a process. So take heart and be light with the self-criticisms when you have relapses in working to recover your body. It is the nature of how people change that recovery is a spiral path, not a linear one. Give yourself permission to begin anew, as if there had been no beginning before. Each stage can be entered into for the first time, unclouded by previous failures, if you allow yourself to see it that way.

I have a client who loves to play solitaire. What she loves about the game is that every game is a new beginning. It doesn't matter what happened in the previous games. With every new hand, she has a fresh chance at winning. History makes no difference. I urge you to consider adopting this winner's attitude as you begin each new "hand" of these exercises.

Before you start, I would like to give a few words of warning about this book. The first warning is of a psychological nature. The exercises in this book will bring up emotions. They are designed to do that, to help you connect to your emotions again through your body. If at any point you feel that something is happening that you do not want, just simply stop what you are doing. There is no requirement that you have to make yourself endure what you feel unprepared for or are unwilling to experience at this time. There is nothing wrong with deciding you do not want to do something suggested. It doesn't mean anything. You win no points for virtue by enduring what is unbearable. Many of you have spent too much of your lives doing that already. Stopping may be the best way of taking care of yourself. I encourage you to stop short of "losing it" or becoming overwhelmed. Take good care of yourself and stop when you feel you've done enough. It may take you months or years to get to all the exercises in this book. Some exercises you may never opt to do. That's fine. You may never meditate on a daily basis. I do because I need to for my own sense of well-being. Recovering your body is not dependent upon doing every exercise in this book. Your recovery begins when you take action to recover. Any of the exercises in this book will start you on the path. I have organized them in an order that makes sense to me. There is no precise formula or timetable that has to be followed. Take your time and do what's right for you. It's your life and your recovery, and you have the rest of your life to work on it.

Don't judge your progress by comparison to anyone else or even by comparing yourself to your own expectations. There is no "right" way to recover your body any more than there is a right way to sleep. Eight hours a night is recommended, but we all know that sometimes we need more sleep and sometimes we can get by on less. Our bodies do what they need to do when they need to do it. There are two right things, though, that you can do for your body to help it recover. One is to set aside daily time, even five or ten minutes, to do a body-recovery exercise. Nothing can happen if you don't allow space in your life for it. The other "right" thing to do is to give your body what it needs, not what it wants. The more you recover your body, the more you will be able to distinguish between the two. What I need at any moment in time may have nothing to do with what you need or even what I need at another time. So skip the judgments as much as you can. You will do these exercises in your own way—not right, not wrong—just how *you* do them. Just do them, at a snail's pace, with a steady jaunt, or an all-out sprint. There is no race. Do them in such a way that you can sing, like Frank Sinatra, "I did it my way."

If you are in therapy, you may want to try the exercises with your therapist before you do them on your own. They are designed so that someone else—a friend or therapist—could read you the instructions and guide you through it. Trust your intuition and do what seems best for you.

Taking good care of yourself also means not pushing your body beyond your own safe limits. While this is not a book for physical conditioning, some of the exercises in this book are physically strenuous. If you have any concerns, consult with your physician before doing any of the exercises that demand gross physical movements. Above all, be kind and gentle with your body. It has suffered enough already. It will thank you and reward you with increased energy, less physical suffering, fewer illnesses, and an overall sense of well-being that is simply not possible when you live disconnected from the body that carries you.

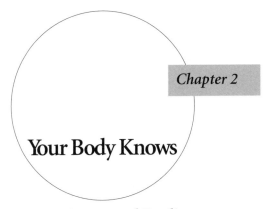

Chapter 2

Your Body Knows

Memories, Experience, and Reality

> "Reality is perceived through your own body."
> —*Vimalakirti Sutra*

Experience, all of it, is a direct knowing through outer or inner senses or both. Reality is what we perceive to be real through our senses. It is only through the body that we can get an experience of reality and can understand the world. When you know something in your body, you know it. Until you know and incorporate it in your body, reality is an abstract concept. The body is the objective experience of consciousness. I could describe to you in great detail the shape, color, texture, smell, and taste of an orange or an orgasm. You might get the general idea, but not until you taste an orange or feel the "petit mort," or "little death," as the French call orgasm, will you know the reality of either one. When you experience, you know.

For the most part, people have a very precise knowing of reality. Yet through dissociation or denial, people discredit reality. On a more or less continuous basis, we all discount or discredit what we experience. We do it with rationalizations, disbelief, and deliberate inattention to our physical experiences. But the body doesn't lie. Our senses connect us to the past. Through the senses, the body experiences, knows, and remembers, no matter how successful we are at consciously forgetting.

My client Sarah, after several years of doing the painful work of remembering the abusive traumas of her childhood, once said to me, "Sometimes this all seems so unreal. I wonder if I made it up." I asked if she wondered that when she had a body memory. She looked shocked. There was no way she could deny the reality of her experience when she thought of what happened in her body when she re-experienced an incest memory. The convulsive terror, nausea, gagging, genital pressure and burning, and the suffocation were feelings experienced with such overwhelming intensity that Sarah knew she could not have imagined them. Body memories cannot be false memories, any more than remembering a song or a smell can be "false." But sorting out the body's memory from the story surrounding the experience can be complicated.

Sarah might have felt more confident of her experiences had she known more about the physiology of memories. Knowing why something happens can be reassuring. Explanations give us a greater sense of control. If the pilot tells us that "we are experiencing some turbulence" when the airplane starts bumping, our fear lessens, at least a little. Because I think it will allow you to feel more secure in handling whatever memories come to you in the process of recovering your body, I want to give you some information about memories, and how they are made, lost, and retrieved.

The area of memory retrieval is fraught with controversy and debate. For starters, there is no agreed-upon definition for "body memory." Illana Rubenfeld, who developed the Rubenfeld Synergy Method for integration of body, mind, and emotions, defines body memory simply as "a holding pattern, the muscles remembering a particular event or series of incidents in a pattern of tension [in response to abuse, injury, illness, shock, fear, anger]." But memory is an extremely complicated operation. Memory doesn't occur just in the brain or in a particular site in the brain. "Memory resides nowhere, and in every cell," says Saul Schanberg, Ph.D., professor of pharmacology and biology at Duke University Medical Center. "It's about 2,000 times more complicated than we ever imagined." The controversy hinges in part on how the brain works, and that miraculous process is still unfolding. More about that process, how memories are thought to happen, will be presented later in this chapter. For the work we are doing here, the purpose of discussing memories is to invite you to be open to whatever you might experience in doing the exercises. It's not necessary at the beginning of this work to judge what's "real" or "not real." As you come more fully into your body, you will know what to trust. The greater risk for those who have been abused is denying the experience.

There has been much controversy in the arenas of both psychology and the law about "false" memories, with psychologists, psychiatrists, memory researchers, and attorneys trying to sort through the complicated maze of what a person actually remembers experiencing and what is a forced or manufactured memory. The purpose of this workbook is not to convince you that some abuse did or did not happen to you. It is to enable you to restore well-being and aliveness to your body. You may have some body experiences and reactions that lead you to conclude you were abused. That conclusion is best drawn with the support and guidance of an experienced therapist. Trust your body. You do indeed feel what you feel in your body. But the body cannot tell you the whole story nor tell you what to do with the story.

I used to be pretty good at denying what I was feeling, physically or emotionally. Now it's not so easy. When I get angry, I instantly feel my jaw and neck muscles tighten and my face get hotter. It's so subtle that I doubt most people looking at me would notice, but I do. It's hard for me now to convince myself that something doesn't upset or excite me when it does. Recovering the body means rediscovering through the senses your own reality, past or present. The reality you reclaim might be forgotten memories of abuse, trauma, or shame, or it may be the reality of what you are experiencing in your life and in your body right now. Waking up to your reality may be global or very specific.

Susan, another client, describes how she reconnected with her body's experiences: "I came to you 'numb,' and off and on I feel numb again, but I know that I am. Overall, I have learned to listen to my body and feel. I feel actual physical hunger, which I really wasn't aware of before. I feel the twinges and the aches and pains. I know when my body is telling me that relationships are bad."

The more you learn to trust the experience of your body, about the past or the present, the more confidence you gain in your ability to know what's real. You also gain an increased awareness in the nuances and cues. Here are some of the things Louise said she learned about her reality through her body:

❍ When I would meet men, I would sometimes get very cold or very hot. I learned that the cold was fear and hot was lust. The latter was not so surprising. Now I notice when I'm feeling unusually cold and realize that I'm fearful.

❍ When I meditate as I walk, I increase my peripheral vision. Conversely, when I obsess while I'm walking, my peripheral vision decreases.

○ When I think obsessively, I feel as though the brain cells in the top of my head are red and swollen. When I meditate, I feel my brain cells go back to normal.

○ When I am fearful, I have a lot of diarrhea.

○ My neck gets a little stiff when I'm being inflexible. It clears when I become more flexible about the issue that I'm concerned about.

○ During incest memories, I become very red-faced and sexually aroused. I also get a certain unusual look on my face, a contorted look, that I never get any other time. I can't mimic the look.

○ Before the memories of the abuse started to occur, I would grind my teeth more than now.

○ When I don't feel strong enough to handle what I need to do, I become more hungry and gain three or four pounds. It's usually a sign to me that I am doing too much and need to nurture myself.

○ I get vaginal discharges when I obsess negatively about my husband and have sex anyway. If I start thinking positively about him, the discharges vanish without antibiotics.

○ My immune system is weakened when I get stressed. I will have cold-like symptoms; my pierced ears will be slightly infected; and I might have a slight vaginal discharge. If I nurture myself by resting, these symptoms go away.

Louise is describing the reality of her body. It may be similar to or not at all like yours. The point is that she has learned to trust her body's experience and to count on it to help her understand what happens to her physically when she has certain mental or emotional responses. The more you trust your body's experience, the more you learn about your own reality and the more you'll trust your body. This circle, when followed repeatedly, leads to greater and greater recovery of your body, and confidence in your ability to know your own unique pattern of responding.

Doesn't everyone know this already? In a sense, yes. We do know how our bodies are reacting to our thoughts, to feelings, and to life events. What varies widely is the extent to which people are consciously aware of their bodies' responses. People say, "I just have a gut feeling about that" or "I can feel it in my bones." We do know, but sometimes we don't want to know. Being present in the body can be too much at times. Psychological or even physical survival may depend on not knowing and feeling the reality of what is happening to us. Sometimes we need to forget.

There is a psychiatric condition called alexithymia. People who have this condition make no connection between their body sensations and their emotions. They can't feel love for people, or any other emotion, because they have such a complete separation of their physical responses from what they experience happening to them. When a person is cut off from the awareness of physical responsiveness, it's simply not possible to know that someone makes your heart beat faster or that a piece of music moves you to tears. I feel very sad for people with that condition. It must be like being a mummy in a tomb. How did they get that way? Probably the same way everyone loses their body to a lesser degree: It was a matter of survival.

No matter what we do to forget, physically some, if not all, of our memories do remain. But those memories are lost to consciousness for many reasons. Children as young as two years old report memories from even months before. Yet few of those memories are retained into adulthood or even into the next year. One reason for the forgetting may be that toddlers acquire the skills for remembering significant events in their lives only when they have the developmental ability to have conversations with others about those events. For most children who are abused, there are no conversations about the abuse that is happening to them. A child sexually assaulted in the night wakes in the morning to be asked, "Do you want cornflakes or pancakes?" There is no way for the child to make sense out of what happened, except to forget that it ever happened at all.

Some memory researchers suggest that we are unable to remember traumatic events that take place early in life because the hippocampus, the part of the brain that plays an important role in processing complex information and declarative or "story" memories, has not matured enough to form consciously accessible memories. Even so, the emotional memory system, which may develop earlier, stores these memories somewhere in the body. The unconscious memories are there and may show up in behavior and emotions even though they are inaccessible to the consciousness.

"Memory is influenced not only by previous knowledge but also by events that happen between the time an event is perceived and the time it is recalled," says Robert Ornstein, Ph.D., author of *Evolution of Consciousness: The Origins of the Way We Think*. What comes to conscious recall, then, is influenced by so much more than the actual events. He says, "So our memories, as exact, recorded, fixed images of the past, are an illusion." I believe this is true of what is remembered cognitively, but the body's recall may be something different from cognitive retrieval. There is a plethora of sound scientific evidence that memories are stored in the body. The body and brain don't forget, even when there is confused or incomplete mental recall. Cells have memories. A person's whole history and deepest feelings are recorded, to be seen, read, and remembered in the body.

Oliver Sacks, the neurologist-author who wrote the book *Awakenings,* about his work bringing post-encephalitic patients temporarily back to aliveness with the drug L-DOPA, tells a wonderful story of taking one of his patients, "Greg," to a Grateful Dead concert. Greg was an amnesiac with a brain tumor and no coherent memories of life since about 1969. But Greg had an encyclopedic memory of the years before and a passion for the Grateful Dead music.

When Dr. Sacks took Greg to the concert, he was enchanted by all the early music and not at all amnesiac. During the second half of the program, when the band played their newer songs, Greg was simultaneously bewildered, frightened, and enthralled. Sacks tried to keep the new memories fresh, but by the next day, Greg had no memory of the concert. All of it seemed to be lost. "But," says Dr. Sacks, "and this is strange—when one played some of the new music, which he had heard for the first time at the concert, he could sing along with it and remember it."

How could that happen? Obviously, there are still many mysteries and miracles of memory. For us to understand how the body may hold our memories, not just those of emotional or physical trauma, it is necessary to understand a little of how memories are made. The whole field of memory research is complicated and rapidly expanding, and there is no precise, definitive explanation of exactly how we remember, but some understanding of different types of memories and the processes in the brain can help. Even though understanding memories is complex, I urge you to read this section. Knowing more about what is happening to you will help, especially at times when what you're are experiencing makes no sense logically.

One type of memory is called declarative memory. These are memories we draw on when we remember what happened to us and how we experienced it. They are thought to be "laid down" differently in the brain from emotional memories, which I will discuss shortly. Declarative memory involves explicit, consciously accessible material. I can remember going to my pediatrician Dr. Bickel's office, wheezing as my mother and I watched the doctor's white cat cruise around the waiting room, being called into her examining room, and making my body rigid by squeezing a penny my mother had given me while I felt the painful sting of the gamma globulin shot in my bottom. This declarative memory was mediated by the hippocampus and cortex parts of my brain. It has a story, and I can recall it consciously.

Dr. Joseph LeDoux, a professor of neural science and psychology at New York University, believes that, in contrast to declarative memories, "emotional learning that comes about through fear conditioning is not declarative learning. Rather it is mediated by a different system, which in all likelihood operates independently of our conscious awareness." That different system involves the amygdala, an older part of the brain, which seems to release emotional responses before we completely recognize what it is we are reacting to or what we are feeling. My body was responding with fear, an emotional memory, as soon as I began to get sick, long before the doctor's nurse brought in the shot, because the amygdalic system of my brain had a learned response of connecting wheezing with getting a painful shot. Says Dr. LeDoux: "Emotional and declarative memories are stored and retrieved in parallel, and their activities are joined seamlessly in our conscious experience. That does not mean that we have direct conscious access to emotional memory; it means instead that we have access to the consequences—such as the way we behave, the way our bodies feel. These consequences combine with current declarative memory to form a new declarative memory."

Emotional memories can be activated by any stimulation of the senses. All the senses go from the organs and then to the brain. Dr. Candace Pert, an internationally recognized pharmacologist, says memories are not just in the brain, although the hippocampus is critical as a gateway in accessing memory. There are ganglia, masses of nerve cells, on the outside of both sides of the spinal cord that squirt out peptides—molecules made up of chains of amino acids that are brain messengers—which go up to the brain and down to the organs. We have different memory states, depending on what peptides are released and received by the peptide receptors. Dr. Pert suggests that if the information being received by the central nervous system is too overwhelming for the brain to handle, as it might be with psychological or physical trauma, the peptides may bounce back down and be stored in the tissue of the body. Somatic tissue (muscles, organs, nerves, ligaments) then serves as a storage facility for memories. So the senses of sight, sound, smell, hearing, and touch may evoke memories that would not arise otherwise.

Dr. Bessel van der Kolk, a psychiatrist and assistant professor at Harvard, who has done extensive research on traumatic memories in incest survivors, says, "The body is a much better scorecard than the mind. The body keeps reacting as if the trauma is happening over again." This is called state-dependent learning, which means that the "state" of the body at the time of the trauma is reactivated. These memories are not repressed, in the sense of the unconscious's not wanting them to surface. Rather they are emotional memories, recorded in the brain and body in such a way that they cannot be consciously recalled.

Dr. van der Kolk has found that it's not just memories of actual experiences of abuse survivors of childhood trauma don't/cannot recall. Incest victims often have poor memory for everything that happened in their lives during the time of their abuse. They have very global autobiographical memory impairment. Their whole past is one big mush. Many can remember nothing before a certain age. The extent of the global memory impairment is a function of the severity of the trauma. If there was continuous child abuse that pervaded every aspect of the child's life, the memory impairment is severe. Reclaiming those memories is a long and painful process, which working with the body will facilitate. But, as Dr. van der Kolk says, "Some experiences are too horrible to ever be remembered. The tale cannot be told without the heart breaking. A cover story is needed." The cover story may be one that goes like this: "I don't remember anything before age seven and my life is a mess, but I came from a loving family and had a happy childhood." If missing pieces of your history don't come back, take what comes and leave the rest alone for now. The unconscious has great wisdom in knowing how to protect us. You will remember what you need to remember precisely when you need it.

Once sensorimotor emotional memories come up and are acknowledged, gradually more pictures and body memories come. The fragments become larger, and the connections get filled in. Dreams may bring memories. There still may be no words, and the person can start to feel crazy at this point. The images may snowball, or slowly a conglomeration of images starts to make sense. But there is a natural reluctance to remember more. We all have a hard time remembering what is alien to us. As one woman put it, "I felt as if I was on an express elevator to hell." People don't want to believe they were sexually or physically abused or to remember mind-shattering traumas. This is when it is vital to have the support of a good therapist who can help you contain the retrieval process as you go through it and help make sense of what you are experiencing.

Understanding the difference between declarative and emotional memories can be helpful in trying to understand what may be happening when you have a body memory or flashback. A flashback is the term given to a sudden memory fragment and/or intense emotion triggered by external cues without one's conscious control or awareness.

It is now possible to see pictures of the brain remembering. The pictures show that the memories of what is known but forgotten occur in the part of the brain that is responsible for seeing, not thinking. It is as if the pictures of the memory are stored in some forgotten photo album. We don't think about the events until we see the picture. Then the emotional memories may come rushing back. The body responds with a memory without any conscious awareness of the trigger. People can have flashbacks, or whole-body recall, and not know what happened to cause them, because an emotional memory with no declarative memory has been accessed.

Flashbacks happen to all of us. Smell, taste, touch, sight, sound can all unleash memories. "Hit a tripwire of smell, and memories explode all at once. A complex vision leaps out of the undergrowth," says Diane Ackerman in her book, *A Natural History of the Senses*. Helen Keller, who suffered great psychological anguish in her early life because of the loss of both hearing and vision, had an exquisite understanding of the power of smell to take her back. "Smell is a potent wizard that transports us across thousands of miles and all the years we have lived. The odors of fruits waft me to my southern home, to my childhood frolics in the peach orchard. Other odors, instantaneous and fleeting, cause my heart to dilate joyously or contract with remembered grief." For Charles Dickens, "a whiff of the type of paste used to fasten labels to bottles would bring back with unbearable force all the anguish of his earliest years, when bankruptcy had driven his father to abandon him in a hellish warehouse where they made such bottles." So flashbacks can be rewarding or painful. When what comes crashing back are remembered experiences of abuse or shame, flashbacks can be traumatic and terrifying. Author and Presbyterian minister Frederick Buechner reflects, "We never really forget anything, they say, and all our past lies fathoms deep in us somewhere waiting for some stray sight or smell or scrap of sound to bring them to the surface again. Those intentionally-forgotten pasts resurface sometimes suddenly and dramatically."

One dramatic example of a flashback's being triggered by a visual memory is illustrated in the experience of Eileen Franklin. Ms. Franklin wrote a book called *Sins of the Father*, in which she recalled remembering, twenty years later, her father murdering her eight-year-old friend. In 1989, Mrs. Franklin was playing with her five-year-old daughter. Suddenly, the look on her daughter's face and a certain way the child's head was cocked triggered a memory of the childhood horror. What Ms. Franklin saw was her father's silhouette. He was holding a rock over his head and brought it crashing down on her best friend's head. The look in her friend's eyes at the moment of her death had been the same as the one Eileen saw in her own daughter's face twenty years later. Her best friend, eight-year-old Susan Nason, had been brutally murdered in an unsolved crime in 1969. Eileen Franklin's father was subsequently convicted of first-degree murder. (That conviction was overturned by a Federal judge in 1995 because of errors by the lower court regarding the admissibility of evidence.)

It is not necessary to have witnessed a murder to block painful memories and to be holding them in your body. The smell of oranges and cloves brought back intense pain and shame for a friend of mine. When she was five, she made her mother a Christmas gift. It was an orange that she had painstakingly studded with cloves. My friend was thrilled with her loving creation and could hardly wait until her mother opened the red cellophane on Christmas morning. Her mother, who was pregnant at the time, opened the wrapping, exclaimed, "What is that disgusting smell?!" and threw it into the trash can. No other word was ever spoken about the gift. The little girl locked the pain, shame, and grief in her body. Smell unlocked the poison of the words.

The poet Maya Angelou knows about the staying power of words. "I do believe that words hang somehow in the draperies and settle in the upholstery and help polish the furniture, go into the clothes—really—and then go into the body, as effect. So they cause us to be well and hopeful and happy and high-energy and wondrous and funny and cheerful. Or they can cause us to be depressed. They get into the body and cause us to be sullen and sour and depressed and, finally, sick."

Music, like words, can trigger memories. Actress Lynn Redgrave, performing in *Shakespeare for My Father*, a production she wrote as a tribute to her father, Sir Michael Redgrave, tells this story of being thrown back to childhood anguish by music:

"And when the call came to tell me that my father died I was expecting it. I'd seen him three weeks before in the hospital in London, but now I was back in New York rehearsing a play. He died one day after his seventy-seventh birthday, on March the 21st. 1985. In the hospital. My brother Corin with him. Just stopped breathing. I made arrangements to take a couple of days off and fly back to London for the funeral. On the morning I was due to travel, I awoke early as usual in my little loft bed in New York, limbs like lead. And I turned on the radio. Vaughan Williams' 'Fantasia on a Theme by Thomas Tallis.' And suddenly I was a child again, he had come home. Fear. Pain. Rudi, Daddy's horrifying brown and white bull terrier, is hurling himself at me as usual, knocking me backward onto the flagstone path. I let out an ear-piercing scream, 'Help!' Daddy rushes out down the steps, picks me up, takes me into the dining room, and spanks me. 'Stop screaming. No wonder the dog gets excited, you're always screaming. Stop!' Daddy is coming for the first time to see me in a school play. I'm Duke Theseus in *A Midsummer*

Night's Dream. I'm fifteen, I'm really nervous. I fantasize about Daddy's post-performance comments. 'Brilliant, Lynny!' 'I never knew you were so talented!' Miss Borchard, my teacher, puts her head around the dressing room door. 'Your father's in front. Middle of the fifth row.' The stained blue velvet curtains on our little stage part, audience murmur quiets, just a few squeaking chairs. My arms are around Harriet, who's playing my Amazon Queen. 'Now fair Hypolita, our nuptial hour draws on apace.' The scene is playing really well. My voice feels strong, so manly. During the first Titania scene, I peek through the curtains to see how Daddy is reacting. His seats are empty. In my loft bed I started sobbing out loud. And then it was gone as quickly as it had come, leaving me shaking and exhausted. That's really odd, I thought, because up until now my grief had been for him, for the loss of his talent, for its effect on Mum. Not for myself." The music lanced the boils of painful memories.

Children who have been physically, emotionally, or sexually abused have to learn to numb themselves in order not to feel the words, touches, or emotions. They dissociate to shut out the pain. To feel all the pain would be overwhelming and mind-shattering. That loss of contact is intentional. There is a lifesaving need not to experience the feelings, sensations, and memories. Imagine, for a moment, what happens to a child who is being sexually abused. I will describe what it was like for one of my clients.

Her eyes flew open as she heard the solid footsteps on the stairs. As a shadow broke the light under the threshold, her small body stiffened and her breath stopped. Slowly, as the doorknob turned, she pulled into a tight ball and shut her eyes. If she didn't move at all, maybe he'd think she was asleep and go away. Maybe. Or just kiss her "goodnight," like he did sometimes. She felt his enormous body as he stood near her bed. The flowered sheet was a hopeless shield. When his boozy breath hit her face, she dug her nails into her tiny palms to keep from throwing up or screaming. No sound came from her clenched throat as he touched her leg. No breath movement of her belly or chest broke her rigidness. Then somehow she no longer felt his hands or his mouth on her. Not any part of him. She didn't feel anything, anywhere. Her body moved, but it was not her moving. No, she's somewhere else, not in that bed, not in that body. She went where there was no pain, where nothing bad was happening to her.

This child dissociated to save herself, just as you may have. But it is not only those who have suffered childhood abuse who dissociate. I want to explain a little about dissociation so that you will think about your own ways of dissociating—how and when you lose your connections with your body. Dissociation, or disconnecting from our experiences at times, is something everyone does. Dissociation can be on a behavioral, emotional, intellectual, physical, or spiritual level. We dissociate behaviorally when we do something without being aware of doing it, like putting our keys down and not remembering where we put them, or putting something in the shopping cart that we had already put in a few minutes before. On an emotional level, everyone shuts down on feelings sometimes and only later lets loose with the tears or anger. I believe that is one of the reasons the headache medicine industry is such a success. Painkillers keep us from knowing how much we may need to scream or weep, which, admittedly, isn't always practical to do as soon as we feel it.

Scarlett O'Hara, in *Gone With the Wind*, knew how to dissociate on an intellectual level. When, as she surveyed the wreckage of her life, she uttered her famous "I'll think about that tomorrow," Scarlett was deciding to dissociate intellectually. More serious dissociation is amnesia, the condition in which people forget parts of their lives or even who they are.

So great is our capacity for physical dissociation that, following an accident, people have been known to crawl or walk long distances for help before registering the overwhelming pain of their injuries. That's a very direct way dissociation can save our lives. Dissociation from the body also can be a form of psychological coping. One of the findings of the Harvard Project on Women's Psychology and Girls' Development was that girls, as they move into adolescence and begin negotiating young womanhood, experience increasing disconnection from their bodies, from embodied information received through sensation. Many young girls seem to quit listening to their bodies in order to be able to adapt to what they perceive society expects of them. That young women are choosing to disassociate from their bodies is a tragic loss for them individually and for us as a society.

Transpersonal dissociation is experiencing no connection with a higher power or a spiritual dimension of life, nothing bigger than self. The continuum of awareness on any of these levels goes from full awareness, which probably no one has all the time, to suppression, denial, repression, and then dissociation.

Thinking about this, you may realize that you disengage in different ways at different times. One woman who had been incested as a child said of her body's numbness, "It's not a matter of dancing on mechanical legs. I have no legs." For you, it may not be this severe, or it may be worse. You may have times when you feel nothing. I have a client who went skydiving because she wanted to "feel something, even fear." It didn't work. She felt just as numb jumping out of the plane and falling through the sky as she had sitting at her desk. All forms of dissociation are protective or coping mechanisms. Dissociation protects from overwhelming trauma and emotions that cannot be integrated into consciousness or daily life. We need it when we are confronted with more than we can handle at any one moment. Everyone has pockets of ignored feelings and body memories. We all have times when we are not fully present to ourselves. That's just the nature of living. The problem comes when too much of someone's life is spent "away from home."

The child who lay in bed listening with fear for the sound of her father's footsteps experienced denial as well as dissociation. Denial is "a primitive and desperate unconscious method of coping with otherwise intolerable conflict, anxiety, and emotional distress or pain." Denial can be about the significance of an event or even about an actual occurrence. When you go from feeling "this can't be happening to me" to "this didn't happen to me," that's denial. When denial and dissociation are combined as a coping strategy, a person becomes "numb and dumb." Denial intensifies with dissociation. It's easier to deny the existence or significance of an experience you don't feel.

The reason dissociation and denial are important for you to consider is that they result in diminished self-awareness and the consequent loss of aliveness. Everyone knows someone who is dead, although walking, talking, and somewhat breathing. Those people look as if they are in suspended animation. Their eyes are dull and nonresponsive. No one's home. They have lost contact with the body that carries them and have stopped knowing what they want or feel. They no longer feel sustainable joy or pleasure from the body. When your pleasure has been blighted, only the blight may be remembered or bodily pleasure may be contaminated with suffering.

Pictures help me to understand. Seeing a diagram of the different responses to stimulation may be helpful to you. E. W. L. Smith, in his book, *The Body in Psychotherapy*, gives a model of a healthy cycle of response to awareness of pleasure and pain. He calls it the Contact-Satisfaction-Withdrawal Cycle (see figure below). The cycle begins when you have a want or need—for food, touch, or whatever. The want or need produces a physiological arousal. If the arousal is strong enough, you become conscious of it. This conscious awareness is experienced as an emotion, longing, revulsion, fear, eagerness. All this happens internally, with no external expression up to this point. You aren't doing anything, but you have feelings about what is happening inside you.

If the experience of the emotion is not blocked by denial, dissociation, or a conscious decision, some movement or action naturally results. You experience hunger and go to the refrigerator for food. You ask for a hug or tell someone he made you mad. If the interaction between you and the environment is successful

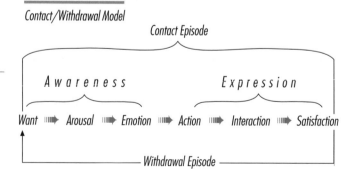

Contact/Withdrawal Model

(e.g., you get some food from the refrigerator or get the hug), there is some satisfaction of the want, and you can go on to the next task in your life. Mission accomplished. But when the want is kept from awareness and/or expression, you are left feeling a tension. If you repeatedly don't express your want or need, as is the case in abusive or shaming situations, you build up an enormous backlog of unfelt and not-acted-upon emotions. The holding back can be painful physically as well as mentally. When you express what you need in some way, you relax. Sarah's experience in a psychotherapy session with me illustrates the point.

Sarah, who had been seeing me for several years, began the session confused and sleepy. She couldn't seem to figure out what she wanted to talk about or work on, and she was really struggling to stay awake. I listened for a while, long enough for me to get confused and sleepy. Finally, I asked, "Sarah, what do you need?" "I need to lie down and be held." We moved from our respective chairs to the massage table in my office. I sat on it, while she lay down with her head in my lap. I had to stroke her back only a few minutes when her thoughts began to flow and she talked easily about what was most on her mind. Soon she sat up, we finished the session, Sarah left energized, and I felt clear. Often it doesn't take much to get our wants met. Verbal expression may be enough for satisfaction. But if you do nothing, you can't cleanly move on.

To hold all those emotions back requires coping

strategies. Denial and dissociation are two. Addictive behaviors are another. The more you block a natural expression of an emotion, the less and less self-aware you become. As one of my clients observed, "I used to dissociate to get away from pain. Now it's beginning to be painful to dissociate. It's a painful separation." To be aware necessitates feeling those wants and risking their expression. Food, drugs, alcohol, sex, work can all help block out feelings—for a while. But those "blockers" cause complications in our lives. When the complications get burdensome enough, people try to get their addictions under control. The problem is that they may get one addiction under control only to find themselves struggling with another addictive craving. The tension, the unexpressed actions and feelings, have to be released in some way or the physical and emotional pain remain. The exercises in this book can help you release those tensions in a safe way so that you don't have to block your experience of living.

One way you may be blocking the experience of your body is with medication. Millions of people turn to medication for relief from emotional pain stored in the body. Eighty percent of the American population swallows a medical prescription every twenty-four hours. Perhaps as long as there have been medicine men and women, shamans, curanderas, and healers of all sorts, people have sought them out for relief from pain. Treatments often include or consist entirely of ingesting something, some medicine. Medicines do work. Many times the pain does go away. The success of the pharmaceutical industry is testimony to that fact. But no pill can free us from pain or deliver a sense of peace without a price. Chemical treatment of anxiety is an example.

Four to 7 percent of Americans have panic attacks, which are intense anxiety in a concentrated dose. You may be one of them. Almost 11 percent of Americans take antianxiety drugs, mostly benzodiazepines. There are several serious side effects to this medication, including impaired memory. One physician describes Xanax, the most common treatment for panic attacks and the drug most often prescribed for ordinary anxiety that anyone might experience during a rough time in life, as a big eraser that "wipes out people's attention to things." There is also evidence that the beneficial effects of the drugs wear off over time and that the anxiety symptoms may be worse when someone tries to go off the medicine than they were before treatment began.

This is not a condemnation of Xanax or any other prescribed medicine that you may be taking. We can feel grateful for the suffering it alleviates. The problem comes in automatically thinking that every physical pain should be responded to chemically. Only a short stint of television watching will amply demonstrate how conditioned we are to associate physical pain or discomfort with taking something to make the problem go away.

Headaches, colds, backaches, constipation, arthritis,

sore muscles, itching eyes, coughs—all this valuable evidence the body offers us that something is amiss can be obliterated with the "most effective remedy." While the immediate relief from pain offered by using medication is tempting, the body recovers only temporarily and the opportunity to learn from the pain is lost. Be as brave as you can in facing your body's experiences and memories head-on. Don't betray your body or yourself by ignoring or blotting out what it feels and what you remember. Lasting, non-chemical, non-addictive freedom from that pain may be your prize. Even if some physical pain remains, by learning to identify and release blocked emotional expression, you will recover a sense of physical aliveness and peace that can transform the experience of that pain.

Trust what comes to you at least enough to investigate. Artist Louise Bourgeois gives us the encouragement and advice to do that. She declares: "I need my memories. They are my documents. I keep watch over them. They are my privacy and I am intensely jealous of them. Cezanne said, 'I am jealous of my little sensations.' To reminisce and wool gather is negative. You have to differentiate between memories. Are you going to them or are they coming to you? If you are going to them, you are wasting time. Nostalgia is not productive. If they come to you, they are seeds for sculpture." Be jealous of what comes to you, in your body and in your memories.

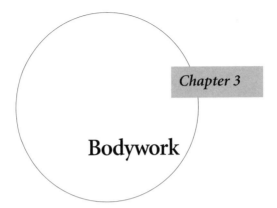

Chapter 3

Bodywork

What it is, Why do it, Whom to choose

"A body who has lived a long time accumulates debris.
It cannot be avoided."
—*Clarissa Pinkola Estés*

Bodywork is a general term that covers many approaches to working directly with the body in order to free up buried pain and blocked emotions. Although there were pioneers in the early part of this century who saw the necessity of working with the body as well as the psyche, bodywork is still not an integral part of most psychotherapy. For me, it is essential in working with clients who have been abused or traumatized in any way. The body holds the memories oftentimes more clearly than the mind does, and the body holds the pain. Jungian analyst Marion Woodman observes, "I realize the voice that says, 'I am unlovable' is in the cells. Therefore it is at that cellular level that the transformation has to take place."

Bodywork is not new. *The Yellow Emperor's Classic of Internal Medicine*, written prior to 2598 B.C., discusses it. It is mentioned in Homer's *Odyssey*. Hippocrates and Asclepiades recommended bodywork as a principle form of therapy. Jesus and his disciples healed broken and diseased bodies with touch. For thousands of years, bodywork has been used to relieve tense muscles, to diminish fatigue, and to soften and free up connective tissue and joints. But touch is still not a standard part of healing the body or the mind, even though for some people it may be a prerequisite for complete recovery from abuse and shame.

Marilyn Van Derbur, the former Miss America who publicly disclosed having been sexually abused by her father and who has since become a valiant advocate for survivors of incest, says, "Bodywork was critically important to me. For so many months, my body felt like a huge ghetto blaster with a dozen rock stations all playing together with the volume as high as it would go. I began to realize that my father had made my child body feel too many conflicting emotions. Rolfing (a type of bodywork) was critically important to me, as was massage … bioenergetics. I could list so many ways I tried to bring peace to my body."

Having your body touched therapeutically can help you reconnect with your body in ways not otherwise possible. Bodywork provides a sensorimotor education. When a part of your body is touched or moved by a bodywork therapist, a flow of sensory information is generated. Parts of your body are in pain all the time, and you don't know it, because your neurological system has adapted. When the muscles start to loosen through bodywork, you feel the pain. You become aware of patterns of tensing and holding, restrictive movements, numb or deadened areas, and temperature variations. As muscles, tissue, and bones are manipulated and tension is released, even more information is available. You gain a sensory awareness of what your body is doing and feeling at any given moment. When the tightly held muscles are relaxed, locked-in emotions may be released and you immediately experience the connection.

You experience first-hand how the interaction between the emotions and body tension is circular rather than linear. Pain in your body brings emotions about that pain, and emotions produce responses in the body, sometimes painful ones. My client Fred says of his experience, "As I healed emotionally, I gained more energy. Slept better. As I released the pain of the abuse through therapy, my body pain would go away." A headache includes the feelings that preceded, accompany, and follow it as much as the tightened muscles and constricted blood vessels that cause the physical pain. Dr. Milton Traeger, founder of one widely used method of bodywork, said, "I am convinced that for every physical non-yielding condition there is a psychic counterpart in the unconscious mind, corresponding exactly to the degree of the physical manifestation." Bodywork helps make the unconscious physical and emotional holding more conscious. Deane Juhan, a teacher of bodywork and author of *Job's Body*, sees the bodyworker as a "diplomatic intermediary ... Touching hands are not like pharmaceuticals or scalpels ... They are like flashlights in a darkened room. The medicine they administer is self-awareness."

Barbara came to me with frustrating back pain. With bodywork and psychotherapy, she was able to make the connection between her back pain and conflicting pressures she was feeling from her parents. She was then in college and being pushed by her father to hurry and finish. At the same time, her mother wanted her to be involved in social activities that were more appropriate to someone just starting college. After listening to her dilemma and looking at her physical stance, I said, "It seems to me that your mother is on top of your back pulling you backwards into the past when you were younger, when she had more control and power over you. The top half of your back is being pulled backwards. The lower half is pushed forward. The push seems to be from your father who wants you to get your degree, make money, pay your bills, take care of yourself, and grow up being responsible." Barbara has very strong parents, and their opposing goals for their daughter literally had her twisted in knots. She did some bioenergetic work that day, which entailed lying on the massage table and kicking as if she were kicking away her parents. That one session didn't settle her relationship with her parents for good, but her back immediately began to loosen and continues to improve. Of the session she says, "In the years since that day, I have always been careful to keep these important lessons in mind."

Bodywork is also used to address directly emotional problems, such as anxiety. Dana had terrible anxiety attacks which came fairly frequently and without any warning. When the anxiety attacks first started occurring, she only felt a burning/itching sensation on her palms and on the soles of her feet, but by the time she saw me, she was hyperventilating and felt she couldn't breathe, because of a closing sensation in her throat. Through bodywork, she relived old psychological pain and felt the crushing weight of responsibility that contributed to her overwhelming feelings of choking and suffocation. Dana let go of the pain with sobs, screams, and movement. When it was over, she breathed more freely. Of the bodywork, Dana says, "I have no explanation of why this worked, but it really made a difference to me. Now I feel as though my body is not my enemy anymore. It's a great feeling—very freeing." Once she resolved the psychological issues, Dana stopped having anxiety attacks, even though she has been in very stressful situations since that time.

The power of touch that comes through bodywork

is as valuable as the emotional healing. The importance of touch cannot be overestimated. Without it, people sicken and grow touch-starved. Touch literally keeps us alive. Part of the regular treatment regime for premature babies in neonatal units is massage three times a day. Massaged babies gain weight as much as 50 percent faster than unmassaged babies. They have fewer complications and are more alert, active, responsive, and "better able to calm and console themselves." Dr. Saul Schanberg, who researches touch with animal experiments, draws this conclusion about the importance of touch: "It's ten times stronger than verbal or emotional contact, and it affects damn near everything we do. No other sense can arouse you like touch; we always knew that, but we never realized it had a biological basis. ... We forget that touch is not only basic to our species, but the key to it."

Bodywork helps you remember the value of touch, which you may have almost lost if you've lived in an unrecovered body. It can help you recover aliveness by increasing your awareness of your own sense of touch. To live with numbness of touch is a tragedy. As author Diane Ackerman, in writing about touch, reflects, "But when we lose touch (the dentist gives you a shot of Novocaine; an arm or leg falls asleep from lowered blood supply), we feel odd and alien. Imagine how frightening it must be to lose touch permanently ... to be without touch is to move through a blurred, deadened world, in which you could lose a leg and not know it, burn your hand without feeling, and lose track of where you stop and the featureless day begins." In an unrecovered body, that is precisely how you live. Bodywork facilitates drawing a much sharper line between you and everything else.

What happens in bodywork? That depends on you and on what kind of bodywork you get. There are two approaches to bodywork: (1) non-psychotherapeutic bodywork and (2) psychotherapy which involves bodywork. Non-psychotherapeutic bodywork has the goals of enhancing body awareness, increasing the flow of energy and fluids in the body, and changing dysfunctional body habits. This bodywork is not designed as an alternative to psychotherapy but as a valuable adjunct. Body-oriented psychotherapy, in contrast, uses techniques that are an integral part of psychotherapy to help you understand what feelings you are holding back and why and to facilitate the release of those emotions.

There are many schools of non-psychotherapeutic bodywork. Some are: Structural Integration (Rolfing), Alexander Technique, Feldenkrais work, massage, Traeger work, Aston-Patterning, Bodytherapy (the work of Dub Leigh), T'ai Chi Ch'uan, Yoga, Aikido, Hellerwork, Reiki, and Shiatsu. Some schools of bodywork that are integrated with psychotherapy are: bioenergetics (Alexander Lowen was a pioneer in this country using this approach), Illana Rubenfeld's Synergy Method, Lomi (Rolfing combined with

Gestalt), Hakomi, and Radix.

Bodywork is also divided between what are called "soft" and "hard" techniques. Hard and soft techniques may be used in either non-psychotherapeutic bodywork or as part of the psychotherapy process. "Hard" techniques are those that apply direct pressure on rigid muscles or on the connective tissue that is causing the muscles to be tightly held in a particular position. Rolfing, Lomi work, and Bodytherapy are examples of hard techniques. There may be pain as the pressure of the therapist's hands directly confronts the rigid holding patterns of the client's muscles. The example I gave at the beginning of the book of having an asthma attack during my first bodywork session involved a hard technique. Specifically, the therapist applied strong pressure along the muscles of my rib cage to loosen the fascia tissue which connects the muscles to the skin. When he did so, the muscles moved more freely, circulation improved, and emotional holding patterns were broken up. And it hurt.

For me, the dramatic results were worth the pain of those particular bodywork sessions. But bodywork does not mean "no pain, no gain." Sometimes pain prevents our bodies from learning. "Soft" techniques can be equally effective and don't entail force or painful pressure. On the contrary, many of them are based on the premise that the body needs to be gradually and gently re-educated as to how to move and stand properly. Most of the oriental approaches to the body have this belief (T'ai Chi Ch'uan, Aikido). Yoga teachings emphasize the noncompetitive, nonstraining principle. Students are admonished repeatedly to stay within their own limits and are told that gradually, with time, patience, and continued practice, the body will become supple. The Sanskrit teaching on this is "Na hathat. Na balat." (No force. No harshness.) Feldenkrais work and Traeger work are two other examples of soft techniques that don't use force or harshness.

The bodywork approach you choose depends on your own assessment of what you feel you want or need. There is no one right way to have bodywork any more than there is a one right method of psychotherapy. Actually, if you've done any of the exercises in this book, you've started bodywork. Many of them are included in one school of bodywork or another. But having a therapist work on your body brings a different dimension to body recovery. Another person is helping you to heal your body.

Where is the best place to begin? If you've had no experience with having someone touch your body in a therapeutic way, I recommend starting with massage. Most towns of any size have licensed massage therapists, since there are now many massage schools in all parts of the country. Swedish massage is a basic one to request. It's an overall body rub that is standard in the training of massage therapists and is a technique dating back to the 19th century. In 1813, Per Heurik Luig established the Central Royal Institute of Gymnastics in Stockholm, where he practiced and taught Swedish massage. Swedish massage has now spread all over Europe and America. Most massage therapists are trained in this and other types of massage and can vary their techniques, depending on what you want and feel you need.

Once you are comfortable with having your body touched and are more connected to yourself physically, you could choose any one of the other bodywork approaches. Select what sounds right to you. No one knows what you need for your healing better than your own inner healer. Trust yourself in choosing an approach and a therapist that feel right for you. Certainly it is prudent and necessary to know something about the bodyworker you select by getting references and asking questions as to training, credentials, and what the therapy entails. Credentials are important, but the most important factors determining the outcome of the bodywork therapy are likely to be the person you choose, your confidence in that person, and your own commitment to change.

The identity and reality of the therapist matter greatly. Studies on psychotherapy have found that "the individual psychotherapist is a significant factor in the … outcome … across a wide range of client diagnoses, severities of clients' psychological dysfunctions, levels of therapist experience, and therapists' theoretical orientations." So whom you choose as a therapist, for the body or the mind, makes a big difference in how you experience the therapy and what the outcome is likely to be.

When looking for a therapist, a bodyworker, or a psychotherapist who works with the body, I recommend keeping in mind "the five R's": respect, rapport, readiness, responsiveness, and reputation. You can get clues as to how a prospective therapist fits the five R's from a brief phone interview.

"The 5 R'S"

RESPECT

The most important of the five R's is respect. By respect, I mean the attitude toward life that the therapist seems to hold. That attitude will be manifested in the stance taken toward you or anyone else. A therapist who has a basic respect for people will listen, even in that first phone conversation, to the basics of what you want or need. After the first session, you should go away with a clear sense that you have been heard and understood and that the therapist values you as a person, cares about what you are saying, and wants to help you recover your body. This respect extends to the respect the therapists have for themselves and, in this kind of work, a respect for their own bodies.

Some people, particularly those with boundary difficulties, want to tell their whole story on the phone before they even have an understanding or an agreement with the therapist that he or she will work with them. A therapist who limits that storytelling prior to making an appointment may not be uninterested but rather is establishing appropriate boundaries. There is a way of telling you "no, I can't or don't need to hear any more of what you're saying right now" that still gives you the sense that what you are saying matters. Even when I don't accept a client, I listen to what he or she needs and make a referral based on those stated needs.

Paul Quinnart, author of *The Troubled People Book*, says this about respect: "If the therapist makes you feel worthless, find another therapist. If the therapist seems preoccupied, day dreaming, or dozing, say something or find someone whose mind is on their work."

READINESS

Does the therapist look ready for you? Is the office prepared and orderly, looking as if you were expected, or is there a sense of disarray? Does the therapist personally seem ready? Does he or she seem prepared?

Honoring time agreements is keeping boundaries. Is the therapist ready on time? Does the therapist meet you at approximately the appointed time, and does the appointment end on schedule? Maintaining time boundaries indicates that the therapist has sufficient control of his or her work to be ready for you. There's an old Zen saying: Watch how a person does something and you will see how he does everything. How a therapist prepares for you shows how he or she will be with you in the therapy.

RAPPORT

When I was growing up, there was a redheaded little girl named Janet who lived on the next street. Try as I might, I never liked that little girl. I played with her sometimes. My mother thought it would be nice if I did. Once I even spent the night at her house, and we slept in a big, high antique bed. I liked the bed, but I still didn't like Janet.

Rapport is like that. Some kids we can play with easily, and some we never can. Some people are perfect dance partners, yet with others dancing is always a struggle. For the therapist-client relationship to work successfully, rapport is essential. Bodywork and psychotherapy are very intimate. The intimacy and trust that build in the relationship between you and the therapist provide the structure that allows for personal change to take place. If the relationship is awkward, if the steps of emotional or physical self-disclosure are met with missteps in response, the learning will be limited. As one of my clients said to me, "Your words, body, eyes validated my pain, which changed my pain and how my body felt." The rapport we had was successful.

Rapport is not a matter of right or wrong. There was nothing really wrong with little Janet. Rather it is a matter of how two people hit it off. We know when we have found the right teacher for what we need to learn. If the therapist doesn't feel right to you and there is no rapport, look further. The "right" therapist may not agree with you and may challenge your ideas. That can be necessary. But at some level there must be mutual acceptance and affirmation.

Making the decision about whether or not you are assessing accurately the rightness of the relationship demands a certain honesty. People who have trouble relating in general will have trouble connecting with any therapist, no matter who it is. One of my clients confessed that she had secretly had therapy sessions with fifteen therapists after she first started seeing me. Her ostensible goal was to find a therapist whom she could trust more than me. Most of the therapists she saw only once. She admitted, however, that with those therapists she did see more than once there came a point where she had to put more into the therapeutic relationship, be more honest and self-disclosing, for anything to happen. At that point, she would quit the therapist. This client eventually had to admit, at least to herself, that the problem was with her, not with all the other therapists. Deciding whether or not you have rapport with a therapist includes doing some honest self-examination. The problem may be yours or the therapist's or the chemistry between both of you. If you can't work it out pretty quickly and get some sense of rapport, move on. The healer you need is out there. Keep looking.

RESPONSIVENESS

My idea of responsiveness is the ability to be responsive to life. What I look for is a therapist who seems to have an acceptable level of health in body, mind, and spirit. There are obvious clues. If the person has a body that looks neglected, is grossly overweight or unkempt physically, or if there is a dullness in the eyes, the therapeutic relationship will be limited. Teachers can teach you only what they have already mastered. A therapist who has not made peace with or does not have respect for the body will not be able to successfully lead you to healing in that area. This is not to suggest the only competent therapist wears a size 8 dress or could lead an aerobics class. Health of body has little to do with shape or size. A healthy body looks healthy.

I was privileged to spend a few days studying with Dr. Milton Erickson, a very wise psychoanalyst and hypnotherapist. Dr. Erickson had polio as a child and was in a wheelchair the rest of his life. He was an old man when I met with him (he died a few months later), yet he still seemed healthy in mind and body. His eyes sparkled. He was curious about us and very present to us and our needs. His old, crippled body had nothing to do with his responsiveness to life. Responsiveness also applies to mind and spirit. Does the therapist seem to be alert, attentive, and free enough from depression, agitation, and fearfulness, as Dr. Erickson was? We are all capable of sensing whether someone else is "with it" mentally. Therapists who seem out of it probably live that way or at least are going through a difficult time in their own lives.

Spiritual responsiveness is important. Being responsive spiritually does not necessarily mean that the therapist attends church regularly. But a lack of reverence for life, an absence of spiritual humility, or diminished spiritual awareness limits the healing to what can be done on the human level. The evidence is clear that emotional and physical suffering is often rooted in damage to the human capacity to feel joy and love, to be caring. Therapists who have not come to terms with their own spirituality and fail to see the link between the body, mind, and spirit will be restricted in how they can help you to see the connection.

The healer you choose depends on what you want to learn. The basic requirement for a teacher/therapist is someone who has mastered the fundamentals of what you want or need to learn. By your own individual standards, you need to be able to believe that the therapist you choose meets your criteria of health and responsiveness in the areas of body, mind, and spirit.

REPUTATION

"By their deeds ye shall know them." That old saying gives useful guidance in choosing a therapist. So how is one to learn about a therapist's deeds? New therapists have had less time to establish a successful track record, but still they can give you useful background information on where they did their professional training and with whom. Most therapists who have been in private practice for a while, on the other hand, have had enough satisfied customers to offer them some guarantee of continued income or they would not have taken the risk of going on their own in the first place. But the clients of any particular therapist, no matter how satisfied, may have needed something different from what you need. The fact that someone has the reputation of being a terrific therapist does not mean he or she offers what you are seeking. Recommendations, good or bad, have to be weighed. Reputation isn't everything. Even the most skillful veteran therapist will have had some therapeutic failures and made some mistakes that resulted in dissatisfied customers. But if the work is basically good and done with integrity and honor, word gets around.

These "best" therapists can be the very ones who are the hardest to get in to see. Having to wait may or may not be appropriate. When you know it's time to take action in your life, it makes sense to seize the moment. Using "the five R's," find an available therapist in whom you can have at least some initial faith, and begin. Reputation is important, but it's only one of the five R's. My experience has been that we end up with the teacher we need for the lessons we most need to work on.

Since my first bodywork session more than twenty years ago, I have worked with many different bodyworkers and healers who had greatly varying approaches. Regardless of their approach, I know having bodywork regularly with skillful therapists increases my vitality, relieves pain, and gives me a sense of general well-being. It is so easy to become disconnected from our bodies that I consider it a necessity, not a luxury, to keep some kind of bodywork as an integral part of my self-care routine. Bodywork increases what I know about myself. I agree wholeheartedly (and "wholebodily") with Deane Juhan when he says bodywork helps us "recall that we are living, growing systems and not just genetic blueprints for engines doomed to begin wearing out the moment that they begin running, that we are an interweaving of processes and not just collections of parts, and that those processes are ultimately open-ended and creative, not mechanically deterministic."

It's a good thing to remember.

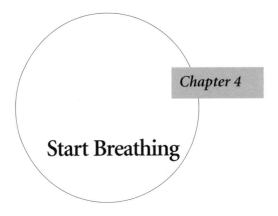

Chapter 4

Start Breathing

"I will sing to you at every moment;
I will praise you with every breath."
—*Psalm 104*

The first step in recovering the body is to *start breathing.* Now that sounds very simple. Of course, we all breathe all the time. But I don't take breathing for granted and haven't since I was a very young child. Anyone who has had asthma or any sort of respiratory disease knows what I mean. Breathing terrified me as a child. The tiny squeak of wheezing that signaled the onset of an asthma attack sent fear through my body as much as any air raid siren. I constricted my breathing in response, which only made my poor alveoli sacs fight more desperately for oxygen. No, I don't assume we all breathe all the time. I know better. With my asthma, I developed an acute awareness of breath. Even if I didn't know what it felt like to take a truly deep breath, I had an appreciation for the simple act of breathing. Most of us do not realize how we breathe and don't breathe.

Breath connects us to life. When breath is restricted, so is energy. Disordered breathing becomes illness, mental or physical. The reverse is also true. When we breathe better, we feel better and actually are healthier. The positive benefits of learning to breathe naturally are immeasurable. Natural breathing has the capacity to calm the agitated body, mind, or emotions. It can energize as effectively as sedate because emotional and physical tension that depletes us of energy can be released through breathing.

One of the first modern-day psychiatrists to understand the relationship of breath and emotions was Wilhelm Reich. He concluded, "There is not a single neurotic person who is capable of breathing out deeply and evenly in one breath." (Reich's follower, psychiatrist Alexander Lowen, was the founder of bioenergetics, an approach to psychological healing that incorporates breath and movement. See Chapter 3.) Dr. Lowen says every emotional problem is reflected in a disturbance in breathing. At Vivekananada Ashram in India, where thousands of people are treated each year with traditional yogic principles for various illnesses, the doctors and researchers have found that the first measurable change with illness is an alteration of the normal breathing rate.

Our body, with innate wisdom, adjusts the breath

to fit our doing, feeling, and responding. Breath, emotions, and actions are indivisibly linked. Breathing changes as emotions change. There is the gasp of air after great sobbing (like a small child who cries so hard he can't catch his breath), the rhythmic breathing of lovemaking, or the slowed breath during meditation.

All too soon, though, children learn how to hold their breath in order to feel less. Tightening the muscles in response to emotional or environmental events and making the breathing more shallow restrict both physical and emotional feelings. The response is automatic. If you are about to be hit, you flinch. Ducking your head protects the chest cavity and covers the heart, and tightening the muscles restricts blood flow and damage to the tissue. It is a natural survival response.

For a person enduring repeated assaults to the body and psyche from physical, sexual, or emotional abuse, the most successful defense is a shutting down of all feelings. The normal response to pain is to react. Reacting normally in an environment that is unsafe can be fatal. Kids learn very early to minimize feelings and to keep from reacting by not breathing deeply. When you start breathing again, very often the feelings that were shut off come to the surface.

Taking a deep breath is one of life's greatest pleasures. The painter Van Gogh knew this when he said, "The fact is that we are painters in real life, and the important thing is to breathe as hard as ever we can breathe." The job of breath in recovering the body cannot be overestimated. Let us begin with the first breathing exercise as a way of demonstration.

Exercise: Watch Your Breath

Please either sit or lie down in a way that is comfortable for you. Keep your eyes gently closed or open, whichever you prefer. Now just breathe normally. As you do so, begin to get a sense of how far down into your body your breath seems to go. Do you feel that it goes just to your nostrils? To your face? All the way to your belly? Does it seem to stop in your throat or chest? Or midway down? Just notice where your breath goes and where it stops. Is it hard to get a breath? Now, with a deep inhalation through your nose, see how far down you can actually pull your breath. Is there a catch somewhere? Or does it just flow on down very nicely and come back up again?

Now see if you can breathe deeply enough to make your belly expand when you take an inhalation. (Do all these exercises with nasal breathing unless you have a cold or are stopped up.) You may want to put your hand on your abdomen to see if your hand goes up when you inhale. The natural way of breathing for little children and babies is for the whole belly to expand. The expansion is below the stomach. Now relax that breath and breathe normally. Try taking three or four belly breaths.

Next see if you can breathe just into your chest,

keeping the breath quite shallow. Do that a few times and compare the difference in sensation between breathing deeply and shallowly. Relax your breath. Then gently open your eyes and sit up if you have been lying down. Breathe normally but with more awareness.

Experiment now with breathing in a different posture. Get up on your hands and knees. If physically you can't do that, just skip this part. When you are on your hands and knees, your back should be flat, parallel to the floor. Your hands are directly below your shoulders. Take a deep breath through your nose, exhaling slowly. Repeat two more times. Then just breathe normally. Notice if it is easier for you to breathe deeply this way. Gravity helps pull down the diaphragm in this posture, which makes it easier for the lungs to expand more fully. This is a good posture to use when you just can't get a deep breath in any other position. Also taking one or two breaths orally can help free up the diaphragm when it's locked.

End this exercise by sitting or lying quietly for a minute or two and invoking a healing Golden Light into the part in you that is now and always will be pure. Take a few minutes to find it. At first you may have some trouble locating that part. Purity is a state, not a place. You may experience it in your heart, solar plexus, belly, between your eyebrows, at the top of your head, anywhere, maybe through your entire body. If you have been badly abused or shamed, the idea of finding a purity in yourself may seem impossible. You may not have any remembrance of your Self and the Whole of you as pure. If that's so, just pretend for now. The experience of this purity will come with time as you repeat the exercise and as you recover your body.

To do this last part of the breathing exercise, imagine a Golden Light flowing into that pure center. You can see the Light coming from an embodiment in which you have faith, such as the heart of Christ, the Buddha, the Omnipresent God, the Holy Spirit, the Virgin Mary, or Brahma. If you don't feel linked to any spiritual Presence, simply imagine the pure Golden Light in front of you, perhaps in the sky. As you breathe normally, imagine this warm Golden Light flowing into your pure center with each breath. Just feel or see the Light come, filling your body with healing energy. The Light is flowing into the pure part of you, the part that will always remain undefiled. Let the breath connect with your purity. As the Light touches and penetrates you, allow it to cleanse and purify all your wounds, pain, suffering, destructive emotions, and shame. Let yourself be dissolved into the Light, even if for only a moment. Rest in this renewing, restoring Light. As the Presence fades, express your "thank you" and go about the business of your daily life, knowing you are now a little different, a little healed.

I will be ending several of the exercises in this book with the Golden Light exercise for applying the healing balm. It is as important as any of the other exercises, maybe more so. Please don't skip it "in the interest of time."

The first thing you may have noticed in doing the breathing exercise is how shallow your normal breathing is. Subtle changes in your breathing will begin as soon as you've done the exercise a few times, maybe even as soon as you take a few good deep breaths into your belly. You might experience unexpected physical or emotional reactions to the simple act of breathing more deeply. Tears may come to your eyes, with or without feelings of sadness. You may start giggling or just feel relaxed. Fragments of memories may surface. Just notice what happens.

Remember back to what it felt like when you shifted from the deep belly breathing to the shallow chest breathing. Were you aware of any difference when you tried to keep the breath in your chest as opposed to having it flow into the belly? Some people feel anxiety or a sense of suffocation when they consciously try to breathe shallowly. Did you discover that you could not get your breath very far down into your abdomen? Was it stuck in your throat or chest? Simply be aware without judgment.

Breathing is the number one tool for recovering your body. Little babies breathe with their whole bodies, unless there has been some trauma in the birthing process or in the uterus. If the umbilical cord is wrapped around the neck or the mother is a heavy smoker, a drug user, or an alcoholic, breathing can be restricted even before birth. But healthy babies breathe freely.

Anxiety and anxiety attacks may be due in part to the experience of breathing difficulty during blocked excitement. A person gets excited about something and needs more air to respond physically to that excitement. The normal, healthy physiological response to excitement of any kind is to breathe more deeply. If the lungs are relatively immobilized by muscular constriction of the thoracic cage, deep breathing is not possible. A panicked sensation results.

Asthma, in contrast, is not a problem of taking in breath. It is a problem of letting it out. Asthmatics can breathe in, but not enough comes out. The lungs don't work very well, and not much exchange takes place. What I wasn't letting out, along with the stale air, was my grief about my father's death. My mother, who had my eight-year-old brother and my eight-month-old sister in addition to me at the time of my father's death, responded to the tragedy with stoicism. Grieving was not an option she allowed herself or us. When I started to have bodywork, the constrictions in my lungs and chest were relaxed. As the bodyworker literally freed my constricted lungs and diaphragm, trapped emotions and memories were released. That long-held grief began to come out. Wheezing, my old defense against the feelings, kicked in.

My client Ann had held her breath since she was

very little. She suffered from severe depression and was persistent in seeking both psychological and physical relief. One evening she sat in a bathtub filled with hot-as-you-can-stand-it water and "detoxing oils": cedar, lime, rosemary, pine. Everything but her face was submerged, and she was miserable. The instruction an herbalist had given her for the bath was to stay in it thirty-five minutes, thirty-five endless minutes to Ann. It hit her, as she struggled to stay in the water, that she had felt this awful feeling before, wanting to get out but not being able to move. Her sweating was the clue to the memory.

As a tiny girl, Ann had climbed under all her covers to the foot of the bed. She lay there huddled, unmoving, and miserably hot. She needed air, but she knew she couldn't come out or move. She was certain something horrible would get her if she came out from under the covers. Ann still doesn't know for certain what would have gotten her had she risked sleeping with her head up on the pillow like her brothers and sisters and other kids. She was sure something terrible would happen, though. Terror kept her paralyzed and trapped. As this memory came back to Ann, she began to choke and sob. As quickly as the feelings began, they stopped, pushed down by some instinctive protective command. She felt ashamed to feel so intensely "for no reason."

Ann switched her attention to her breathing. "I'll just notice how often I breathe. I'll record it," she decided. Ten seconds, twenty, thirty seconds passed before she felt herself needing to breathe. When she did, the inhale was so shallow that the exhalation was almost imperceptible. She kept monitoring. The same pattern continued: more than thirty seconds between barely perceptible breaths. Ann was astonished. How could she possibly be going so long with so little oxygen?

Consciously, with willful intent, she raised her head out of the water and took a long, deep breath. Several times she repeated the almost ritual intake of life-sustaining prana, or breath. Her body began to relax, and a calmness spread through her. Breath had released her from the grip of her terror.

Exercise: Take in Your Share of Air

Try another experiment in breathing. Lie or sit down comfortably. Put one hand on your abdomen, right over your belly button, and put your other hand on your chest, covering your heart. Take a breath with your mouth closed. See if you can make your belly rise up with inhalation. Let the air push your hand out as far as it can. Let go of concerns about not having a flat belly. A flat belly may be stylish, but it's not necessarily healthy. Inhale and exhale a few times. Let the belly expand with each inhalation. See if you feel a slight movement of your chest as the breath is exhaled. Do this for one or two minutes. In and out. You may feel awkward and tempted to judge yourself if your movements do not match the description. Just keep giving your breath a chance. In and out. You may start cough-ing. It's not uncommon that one of the first things that happens with deeper breathing is coughing. Coughing is the body's way of clearing the air passages. Air is get-ting down, and congestion is starting to break up. Allow yourself to claim your birthright of all the breath you need. See how it feels to take in your share of air. If you find yourself struggling and feeling discouraged, just let this easy, deep breathing be a goal to strive for over time. Remember, this is the first step in recovering your body. Breathing is the basic foundation.

Finish this exercise by breathing warm Golden Light into your place of purity for one or two min-utes. Reward yourself with healing, energizing Light for the work of doing this exercise.

Skillful practioners of yoga know a lot about breathing. For more than six thousand years, yoga scripture has taught the importance of breath and breathing techniques for revitalizing the body and calming the mind. Prana is a Sanskrit word meaning "that which moves forward," and every school of yoga teaches pranayama, "restraining or subduing that which moves forward." The techniques are lessons in con-trolling the breath. The purpose of pranayama is to make the respiratory rhythm more regular, which has a soothing effect on the nervous system. Some of those lessons, which have continued through the centuries because of their usefulness, can be very helpful to you in recovering your body. While some Westerners believe yoga is a religion, the word "yoga" actually means "yoke, bind, join, or unify." The breathing exercises offered here, while they may seem strange at first, are for the purpose of unifying you with your energy, calmness, and sense of well-being.

A few concepts need to be explained to help you understand the logic behind the yoga exercises. Modern brain research has shown that the brain functions are divided between the right and left cerebral hemispheres. Each side has its own job. The right brain (which controls the left side of the body) handles intuitive and feeling jobs. The left brain (controlling the right side of the body) is the rational and logical part. The right brain sees pieces as a whole and gives order. Additionally, the right side of the body is called the "pingala," or solar, side. It is the side of us that energizes, heats up, prepares for action. The left side is the "ida," or lunar, channel, the cooling, calming, receptive side. Pranayama lets both hemispheres of the brain "talk" to each other and brings them into balance so that they work together better. The result is the mind's becoming more clear and alert.

The breathing exercises below give techniques for creating such a balance and for energizing/stimulating or calming/sedating your energy when more of one or the other is needed. The second exercise, for example, teaches how to wake yourself up when you are feeling mentally sluggish or sleepy. It offers a means of naturally stimulating the brain without the use of chemicals and can give the benefits of a strong cup of coffee without the side effects of caffeine. The final exercise can be used when it is difficult to quiet or calm your mind. It gives you a chemical-free sleeping potion that you don't even have to buy. These techniques have worked for human beings for thousands of years and will work for you with your conscientious application. I have used them for several years and attest to their effectiveness.

Exercise: Balancing the Breath

Sit erect, in a chair or with folded legs on a cushion on the floor. The important thing is to have your spine erect and to be comfortable enough to sit a few minutes without fidgeting. Close your eyes gently. Put both hands palm up in your lap. Raise your right hand in front of your face, at nose level. Exhale slowly. With the thumb of the right hand, gently close the right nostril. Don't stick your finger or thumb into the nostril. Just use it to press the side of the nostril closed. Now breathe into the left nostril only, keeping the right nostril blocked. Hold the breath. Using your index finger, close the left nostril. Remove the thumb and exhale out the right nostril. Now breathe in the right nostril only. Close the right nostril with the right thumb. Remove the finger from the left nostril and exhale out the left side. Repeat the process for five minutes, breathing in one side, and exhaling out the other. After five minutes, lower your arm, put your hands in your lap, and breathe normally for one to two minutes.

Don't strain in doing this or any of the breathing exercises in this chapter. Breathe naturally, and don't hold your breath in a pressured way. Stop if you feel dizzy or start to pant. If your nose is stopped up, skip this one until it's open again. Doing the exercise can make you feel anxious. If it does, just sit or lie down with your eyes closed until you feel a little calmer. Don't hop up. You'll take your anxiety with you. Do this pranayama exercise once in the morning and once in the evening. The alternate-nostril breathing is said to balance the nadis, or energy channels. It does indeed have a steadying effect. I use it whenever I feel unbalanced or off-center.

Use this next breathing exercise whenever you are fatigued and feeling depleted. It's a quick pick-me-up that can be used as often as you want.

Exercise: Energizing Breathing

Sit upright, spine erect, in a chair or with folded legs on a cushion on the floor. Put both hands palms up in your lap. Close your eyes gently. Raise the left hand and open it, with the fingers pointing upward but touching. Inhale and exhale slowly. With the thumb of the left hand, gently press the left nostril closed. Now breathe deeply only through the right nostril for five minutes. After five minutes, lower your left hand and breathe normally through both nostrils. That's all there is to it. Five minutes of solar breathing and you will feel the difference in alertness and energy. Repeat as needed.

Left-nostril breathing, which is what this next exercise entails, has the opposite effect of the previous one. It sedates and calms you. I use it when I'm having trouble sleeping.

Exercise: Calming Breathing

Sit upright, spine erect, in a chair or with folded legs on a cushion on the floor. Put both hands palms up in your lap. Close your eyes gently. Raise the right hand and open it, with the fingers pointing upward. With the thumb of the right hand, gently press the right nostril closed. Now breathe deeply only through the left nostril for five minutes. After five minutes, lower your right hand and breathe normally through both nostrils. Five minutes of lunar breathing can bring about noticeable increase in tranquility and calmness. You can do this longer than five minutes if you like, but not longer than fifteen minutes. If you're having trouble sleeping, this exercise can be a big help and is much better for you than any sleeping pill.

The recovery of your body has begun! You are on the path. Your job is to stay the course and not falter. Now you are ready to "get moving," which is what the next chapter invites.

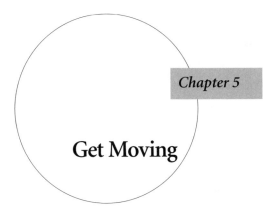

Chapter 5

Get Moving

"How infinite in faculty, in form, and moving!
How express and admirable in action."
—William Shakespeare

Once you have started breathing, the next step in recovering your body is to get moving. Move your body regularly. Two-thirds of Americans do no kind of vigorous exercise on a regular basis, even as little as twenty minutes three times a week. We have become a sedentary nation, and the evidence pours in from many disciplines that we are suffering for it. Movement is medicine. Activity is central to physical health. The scientific data as well as common sense suggests that regular exercise is necessary to function as we are designed to function. I think fear, not laziness, is one of the major reasons people do not move their bodies. People are afraid to start feeling their bodies and the emotions that come with being in the body.

Dance teacher/healer Gabrielle Roth says, "For many of us, the body is a feared enemy whose instincts, impulses, hungers are to be conquered, tamed, trained for service, beaten into submission." Of her own experience as a dancer, she admits: "I learned to ignore, deny, control, misuse and abuse my body. I could make it do fancy steps, rev it up with one drug and knock it out with another, starve it and adorn it, but I didn't trust my body, I didn't like it. No wonder I didn't live in my body, or seldom let my breath move below my neck. Mine became a body disconnected from the waves, the rhythms, the cycles that comprise the ocean of my being. I could dance, but I'd forgotten how to really move or be moved."

My client Sarah, whom I discussed earlier, hated it when she "got moving" in yoga class. It was not the asanas, or postures, that she hated. What she dreaded was the vulnerability she felt when she opened her body and came out of her crouched hiding posture. When she did, fear and shame registered all through her. But Sarah stuck with the yoga classes for many months. When the fear became too great, she would leave class early. Slowly she found the fear lessening. At times she could move with a feeling of security. The sensation of being able to move and breathe without such binding physical restriction was encouraging enough that she kept going to classes. When she would stop for a few weeks, the constricted muscles and paralyzing depression would creep back in. Sarah continues to be pulled between the imprisoning safety of a rigid body and the vulnerable freedom of movement. She doesn't quite long to get moving, but she does move more.

Martha, on the other hand, loves yoga classes. "Tears pour out of my eyes and run all over my face as memories of the pain of my life come back. But I just keep doing the asanas and blow my nose when we change positions." Martha was subjected to incest by her father when she was very small and later, when she was a teenager, by her brother. Her husband beat her, and their marriage was violent almost from the beginning.

When Martha started practicing yoga, she was suffering intense back pain and was often ill with the flu or colds. Her back is much stronger after a year of yoga, and she hasn't been sick in almost that long. Equally important is Martha's increased ability to think clearly. She used to have many accidents (automobile, household) and to be "in a fog." She still makes clumsy, mindless mistakes, like dropping a glass, as we all do. Now, however, she immediately becomes conscious of what is happening and is able to connect it to the feelings and thoughts she was having at the time of the "accident."

All this reconnecting has not been easy in the least for Martha. She is in her forties, and her body has taken the abuse that comes from bearing six children and living with violence. She still forgets her body. "Sometimes I walk out of the house in the morning without ever looking in the mirror. I really don't have any idea how I look. How do I look?" she asks me. On those days, Martha looks like a child without a mother to dress her, or like someone who dressed in the dark. That's exactly what she does on those days: dresses in the dark of her unconscious. The more she does her yoga exercises and the more she is aware of moving inside her body, the less Martha "dresses in the dark." She may never appear stylishly pulled together to others, but she is less likely to walk out the door forgetting she has a body at all.

Author Annie Dillard laments: "We let our bodies go the way of our fears. A teen-aged boy, king of the world, will spend weeks in front of a mirror perfecting some trick with a lighter, a muscle, a tennis ball, a coin. Why do we lose interest in physical mastery? If I feel like turning cartwheels—and I do—why don't I learn to turn cartwheels, instead of regretting that I never learned as a child? We could all be aerialists like squirrels, divers like seals; we could be purely patient, perfectly fleet, walking on our hands even, if our living or stature required it. We can't even sit straight or support our weary heads."

It is life-sustaining and emotionally healing to move our bodies. It's hard to freeze up emotionally if you keep moving. Only thirty minutes of aerobic exercise (fast walking) three times a week significantly lowers the risk of heart disease and reduces depression. Depression loves a still body. For many people, exercise is the only thing that stops a freefall into the abyss of depression. One man who climbed out of that abyss told me, "The one thing I held onto was exercise. I was determined to move my body, even if mechanically, to move my body every day." Healer Caroline Myss muses, "Angels find it easier to guide a verb than a noun. It's hard to receive guidance when you're not moving."

To come back into the body, you have to experience your body's movement. Aliveness has always been associated with action, inner or outer. Without movement, there is not life. Just as there can be a deliberate decision not to move, you must make a conscious commitment to get moving again. Jogging, walking, running, yoga, swimming, cycling, weightlifting, T'ai Chi, dancing will all work. Even if you are in a wheelchair, you can vigorously move whatever you can move. Commitment is the key. There's an African proverb that says, "God will not drive flies away from a tailless cow." We do have to do our own work. Psychologist-runner Keith Jöhnsgard understands the struggle to sustain the commitment to movement: "Whether one is an experienced athlete or a beginner, the problem frequently comes down to taking that first step each day." Once you do commit to taking that first step, be alert, though, to the possibility of making moving a new addiction. The goal is to make a commitment to move mindfully, not compulsively. Movement will bring you back to your body as long as you do not use exercise to go unconscious or to stop feeling. The body may benefit from unconscious movement, but the movement will not serve as a step in recovering the body.

As you begin moving more, you are likely to find yourself moving your body as you move through life in general. I was chased by "Hurry Up," "Be Perfect," and "Be Strong" demons and still am when I lose touch with myself. So it's no big surprise that my movement commitment was running—marathon running. My husband, Blair, and I ran the 26.2 mile courses in New York, Boston, and Houston (all three in a six-month period) with a compulsiveness having nothing to do with loving or being in touch with the body. Despite this determination to conquer my body, I gradually came to know and respect it more. I felt my aching or stinging muscles. I learned to pay attention to my breathing. Eventually I even let my body take the lead in what I would or would not do in training or in running a race.

With awareness, you'll identify old patterns of compulsiveness and excessive use of force and be able to let go of them. When you do this, the physical changes start yielding psychological and emotional changes. The changes that take place in the brain with muscular movement alter the entire body-mind-emotion balance.

Movement is only one of the steps in this book and will not completely overcome all the emotional consequences of abuse and shame, but it can yield quite important benefits, including a reduction in anxiety and rigidities of thinking and feeling. "Movement is the medium of change. In my experience, if you put your psyche in motion it will heal itself. The enemy is inertia, be it of energy in the body, walls around the heart, or fixed attitudes in the mind," says Gabrielle Roth.

You are going to start feeling physically and emotionally much better when you start to move regularly. Perhaps not at first, but it will happen. Give up expecting to feel better immediately after you begin exercising. An average exercise program will give you a 2 percent increase in strength per week. It might be as long as three weeks before you notice any significant changes, but physical and emotional changes do take place if you exercise regularly. Exercise reduces physical tension and reliably reduces anxiety. Mild to moderate exercise produces a predictable general relaxation response whose effects on muscle tension can work as well as or better than a tranquilizer. Listen to your body and use some caution in not letting the psycho-physiological pleasure of exercise become an emotion-blocking addiction. Using exercise to keep from dealing with feelings is not recovering your body. It is substituting one addiction for another. Move mindfully, with awareness and respect for your body.

This first little exercise can help very much in getting moving, even if you haven't yet worked out an exercise program. It's quick, easy, and I think it's fun.

Shake It Up

Stand with feet about six inches apart, spine erect

but not stiff, knees gently flexed. If you have trouble balancing, lightly hold onto a chair back. If you can't stand, do a modification of this while sitting. Raise your right foot. Very gently, shake it a little, like it's asleep and you're trying to wake it up. Do this a few seconds. Put your right foot down. Raise the left foot and give it a little shaking. Put the left foot down. Raise your right foot again, and gently shake your foot and lower leg from the knee down for a few seconds. Repeat with your left lower leg. Now shake your whole right leg, moving it in any direction you want. Do the same with your left leg. Put both feet down. Be aware of the sensation in your legs and how it differs from the rest of your body. Be sure you are breathing while you do this.

Now move the hips. Wiggle them from side to side, forward and backward. Rotate them in a clockwise and then counterclockwise direction. Stop.

Wiggle your shoulders and torso next, shaking them gently like a samba dancer, one forward, one back. Lift your shoulders and let them drop. Wiggle your torso any way that it wants to move. Now stop.

Shake your right hand. Then your left. Shake your right lower arm. Shake your left lower arm. Now shake both arms at the same time. Let them swing wildly or rhythmically. Allow your arms to decide where and how they want to shake and move. Stop for a moment, still standing, and notice how your body feels from your shoulders down. Tingling? Warm? Looser? Be sure you are still breathing as you do all this.

Very gently move your head from side to side. Now let it roll in slow, clockwise circles. Reverse the direction, and roll it in counterclockwise circles. Repeat three times each way.

Finally, shake your whole body all at once all over. You may find some sound coming out of you—a moan, a cry, or even a laugh. Let it come. Shake it all up for a few seconds. Rest. Enjoy the energy you've allowed to flow through your body. This whole exercise can be done in two to three minutes or you can expand it to five or ten minutes.

Notice what you feel. More blood in your head? Maybe you feel invigorated or even numb. Numbness is sometimes a precursor to a more intense sensation. Noting the numbness is a coming back into your body as much as noting any other sensation.

If you regularly sit for long stretches, at work or at leisure, consciously make a decision to move when your body needs to move. Just getting up and walking a little or stretching is part of recovering the body. You can forget that you have a body by getting lost in thought or work. Movement helps you remember. I have a client who routinely doesn't even let himself get up to go to the bathroom until he's finished with whatever project he's doing. It's irrelevant to him that his kidneys or bladder are signaling distress. He ignores the signals, if he notices them at all. That is body abuse.

Regaining confidence in your body's ability to move can be facilitated by remembering how you moved as a baby. This next exercise involves doing some of the first movements your body knew how to do. Approach it with the curiosity of a child.

Exercise: Being a Baby Again

Begin by lying on your back with your knees gently pulled up to your chest. (Modify these instructions to fit what your own body can do.) Wrap your arms around your legs, with your arms either on top of your shins or under your calves. Lower the back of your head to the floor.Close your eyes. Now gently rock your body left and right. Continue the rocking motion for one to two minutes. Let yourself savor the gentle pleasure of rocking.

Then roll over on your side and get up on your hands and knees. Begin crawling all around the room. Crawl fast or slow. Experiment with both. Some babies are never allowed to crawl or to crawl as much as they need. If that was true for you, crawling may feel strange or awkward. Stick with it. Crawl for one minute, letting yourself stop to explore or rest, just as you did as a baby.

Still on all fours, start creeping slowly as a baby does. You might pretend you are very little and sneaking up on a sleeping dog or kitten. Move very slowly.

Notice which arm and leg naturally move together. Creep for one minute.

Come to a kneeling position. Then sit back on your heels. Slowly lower your head forward to the floor, with your back extended straight. Let your arms rest on the floor with your hands palms-up beside the heels. Enjoy resting in the "baby pose," as it is sometimes called in yoga classes. Feel the natural comfort that comes from being "tucked in" and supported by the ground. Sit up slowly after one to two minutes.

Pretend you are a little older child now, perhaps age two or three, four at the oldest. Stand up. Start hopping around the room, both feet together, then on one foot. Hop fast, then slow, then fast again.

Begin to skip. Skip gently, slowly at first. Then change the tempo to suit yourself. Let your arms swing freely. Whistle or sing if you like. Feel the lightness of once again being a little like a child. Feel the pleasure of being inside the body that is *you.*

End this exercise by gently reclining on your back. Let your breathing regulate itself. Close your eyes. Imagine now the warm, healing balm of Golden Light flowing into you. Let it flow into your pure center. If memories or thoughts intrude on the image of the Light, just gently return to Light when you notice you have become distracted. No judgments. Let surface whatever comes. Do this Light-imaging one to two minutes before opening your eyes and getting up slowly.

This much movement can release powerful feelings and memories. Just observe what happens and don't resist. If you feel fear, let yourself feel fear. The same goes for joy, anger, or any other emotion. Jotting down notes about what you remembered or felt can help you make sense of it all as the pieces of the memory puzzle come together.

The next exercise will help you get in touch with how you hold yourself by exaggerating positions and movements. You can do it alone or with others. It can be fun as well as informative.

Exercise: Silly Moving

Begin by doing the worst walk you can imagine. Use every kind of ridiculous posture: pigeon-toed, splay-footed, knock-kneed, bow-legged. Walk around the room trying out each one. As you move, look in a mirror if one is available. Waddle, clomp, and mince. Now make different parts of your anatomy stick out, sag, or flap as you walk. Let yourself laugh at how it feels to move in such an exaggerated way.

Now try to walk your best, an easy but straight balance from your head through the soles of your feet, your weight distributed evenly on both feet, which rest comfortably on the floor. There should be no strain, pain, contraction, or pressure in any part of your body. You may be shocked to find that it is not so easy. Some of those funny distortions are part of your own posture and walk! Don't judge or criticize yourself. Just appreciate what you now know about your "stance in life" and look forward to the changes that will come as you recover your body. Sit or lie down gently. Relax a minute or two, breathing in Golden Light. Remind yourself with the Light that a part of you is perfect and pure, no matter how you walk, stand, or move.

This next exercise illustrates dramatically how our bodies as well as our emotions can be split. It can be funny but also informative.

Exercise: Split Bodies

Stand in front of a mirror, or another person if you have someone who will do this exercise with you. Now practice holding your body and moving in some way for one minute in each of these splits:

- Tight, contracted face with sloppy, slack body
- "Rag-doll" arms and stiff, wooden legs (Try skipping a little in this posture.)
- Happy face and sad body
- Sexy pelvis and "Puritan" face
- Brave chest and scared pelvis
- A man's right side, and a woman's left
- "Yes" with the head, "No" with the hands, and "Maybe" with the feet

Now shake your arms, legs, and head and take

several deep breaths. Lie on the floor on your back. Close your eyes. Take a deep breath. Now quickly tighten your feet, ankles, calves, knees, thighs, and hips. Keep them tight as you take another breath. Tighten your abdomen, stomach, chest, shoulders, neck, head, and face. Tight! Tight! Tight! Hold for two to three seconds. Now exhale forcefully and *relax*. Lie there on the floor, feeling the relief of letting go of the tension and being a "whole" body again. Stay there a few minutes just breathing normally. Breathe in the Golden Light.

Most people feel some, if not a great deal, of self-consciousness when they dance. Don't worry how you look when you move. You bring your history to your movement, and it is an honorable history, no matter what you have done or have been through. Watch your movements through compassionate eyes. As Emilie Da'oud says: "When we watch a seventy-year-old hand move, we feel, 'Yes, that hand has lived.' All the bodies it has touched, all the weights it has cradled are present in its movement. It is resonant with experience, the fingers curve with a sense of having been there ... a truly supple adult movement is awesome, because all of life is included in it." If you can't quite silence the inner critic just yet, do this next exercise for the first time when you are alone. It takes a little preparation in terms of organizing some music before you begin.

Exercise: Dancing Into Aliveness

Pick out several types of music that seem very physical to you. Some possibilities are: hard rock; classical adagios (slow movements) of Bach, Mozart, or Albinoni; Dixieland jazz; Sousa marches; "New Age" floating-type music; Strauss waltzes; folk music; chants (Sufi or Tibetan); Polynesian music; Indian sitar. The important thing is to have a variety of music that will elicit different moods.

Gabrielle Roth has observed that there are "five sacred rhythms that are the essence of the body in motion, the body alive": flowing, staccato, chaos, lyric, and stillness. Flowing music would be the sound of a lonely sax, and the movements to it would be smooth, "only curves, endless circles of motion, each gesture evolving into the next." Staccato movement follows, with music of drums or horns that invite "jerking, jabbing, jamming." Chaos comes when the pace quickens and you are drowned by the beat, about to lose control. Just before you do, a lyrical rhythm takes over, with violins in sweet, fresh tunes. Last comes the stillness, with an inner aliveness.

You might choose to arrange your music according to this pattern of rhythms, or you might choose just to experiment with the music you have on hand or feel drawn to play. Whichever, if possible, put several kinds of music on one tape. It is better not to have to stop to change the music. In any order that suits you, play some music and dance to it. An alternative to dancing upright is to lie on the floor and dance with your body flat and supported.

Let your body go any way the music moves it. If you can, allow yourself freedom to move without being controlled by the inner critical voice. Be aware of any feelings, sensations, or memories that surface to consciousness as you dance, but keep on dancing. See if you can notice what kind of spirit seems to be moving in you—animal, bird, fish, or whatever. We all have animal energy. Free movement in dance helps us to reconnect with it.

Switch to a different music every two to three minutes for fifteen minutes or more if you can. With each new music, move as freely as you can allow yourself to move. Partially close your eyes to see if that helps you feel freer. If you stop to change the music, rest just for a few breaths and dance again. Repeat this process until you have played four, five, or six different kinds of music.

It is *important* that you end with music that is neither angry or sad. You may feel angry, fearful, sad, nor even anguished when you dance. But don't leave yourself there. End with a few minutes of either uplifting or soothing music.

If you let yourself become lost in the music and the experience of the movement, you are likely to find that you have a sense of becoming lighter and moving more fluidly. Enjoy the gift you have given yourself—the gift of free movement.

This is an exercise in dance therapy. Be respectful of the power it has. Plan to do it at a time that will be free from interruptions, and allow for reflective time afterwards. End by lying or sitting on the floor, breathing in Golden Light for one or two minutes.

By the time you have done the breathing and movement exercises in this and the previous chapter, you are well on your way to recovering your body. Don't stop now! There are many discoveries awaiting you, some exciting, some perhaps terrifying, all of them healing. Keep going. The next chapter tells you how to get grounded when you dissociate or space out.

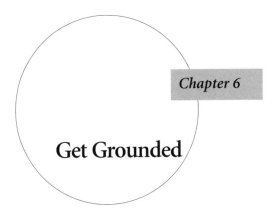

Chapter 6

Get Grounded

"I wonder if I shall fall right through the earth!"
—*Alice in Wonderland*

The definition of ground is "the solid surface of the earth." To ground means "to supply with basic and essential information." If you are not aware of your body, the connection to the earth beneath you is very tentative. You are missing essential information, like where your feet, hands, fingers, and head are in space. You literally may not be in touch with where your body is relative to the earth and objects around you. Stumbling, falling, and bumping into things, you keep painfully discovering that you don't know where you are. Without grounding in the body, it is impossible to know with certainty what you want at any given time—food, sex, rest, exercise, laughter, tears, anger. When you don't keep grounded, what is lost is not just awareness of the body but a sense of being real.

135

How we contact the ground beneath us plays a major role in how solid and secure we feel, not only in moving through time and space but also emotionally. When our contact with the earth beneath us is limited, it's hard to know where we stand, metaphorically as well as physically. The result is an uneasy feeling of continually being off-balance and having to hold ourselves up through sheer will. Letting go would feel like a fall into oblivion. We keep ourselves from plunging into the abyss by raising our shoulders up to our ears, lifting the chin, and relying on intellect. Feet are contracted in fear. It is a terrifying way to have to live and move through life. Our bodies ache from the strain and struggle. I watched Sarah try to hike down a mountain that way.

Most summers my husband and I offer an intensive workshop for my clients. Part of the workshop is hiking up and back down a mountain. These are serious mountains, usually in the wilderness. Everyone has made it up and back in the ten years we have led groups "to the mountaintop." One of our hikers had rheumatoid arthritis. Some were obese. For most of them, this trek was a considerable stretch of their physical and emotional endurance. Sarah has been on two of these climbs with us. On the last one she began to slip and fall as we crossed a snowfield. It wasn't dangerous, but she became very frightened. I watched her stiffen and hold her breath. Her shoulders went up, and her hands contracted into fists. I couldn't see her toes, but I knew they were contracted and clawing inside of her boots.

With each step, she was more and more off-balance. She began to fall every two or three steps.

"Sarah, get out of your head and pay attention to your feet," I admonished. "Feel your toes inside your boots. Feel the weight of your body shifting on the soles of your feet as you step. Feel the ground, the snow, under you. And start breathing." Sarah listened to what I said, took a few deep breaths, shifted her awareness to the sensations in her feet, and didn't fall again.

Like most of you who have lost faith in your body, Sarah doesn't automatically think of turning to hers for support in times of distress or crisis. She stiffens up and gets swamped by thoughts and feelings. This freezing hurts physically and can lead to chronic pain, like the bursitis I had. In addition to chronic pain, when you are ungrounded, your central nervous system is flooded with neurological "chatter" which results from a physiological fear of falling. You may fear or feel like you could easily be "pushed over" emotionally or even physically when this is happening. People who walk around ungrounded to this extent often have difficulty with change. It is like maneuvering through life on stilts. Sudden changes in direction are terrifying when you're tottering so far from the earth.

The cycle is frightening. In response to feeling fear of being out of control, there is an automatic gripping with the toes in an effort to try to "hang on." The problem becomes serious if this pattern is held for years. Contact with the ground becomes chronically limited because contracted feet have a smaller surface for connection with the ground. The less contact the feet have with the surface of the earth, the more off-balance and fearful one feels. You end up lost and afraid. As Buddhist meditation master Joseph Goldstein observes, "As we go through our work, our relationships, our activities, very rarely are we grounded in awareness of our bodies. We're lost in our hopes, our stories, our plans."

Grounding begins by being aware of the entire body. We need to be conscious of what is happening within ourselves when we are still, as much as while we are moving through space and time. Awareness means knowing what we are doing when we do it, and feeling it while doing it. Most of us not only do not know what we are doing, we don't even know that we don't know. I think we all can benefit from the advice given to those who aspire to be Buddhist priests: "A priest in advancing and returning has an accurate comprehension of what he does; in looking and gazing has an accurate comprehension of what he does; in drawing in his arm and in stretching out his arm has an accurate comprehension of what he does; in wearing his cloak, his bowl, and his rakes has an accurate comprehension of what he does; in eating, drinking, chewing, and tasting has an accurate comprehension of what he does; in easing his bowels and his bladder has an accurate comprehension of what he does; in walking, standing, sitting, sleeping, waking, talking, and being silent has an accurate comprehension of what he does."

A starting place for gaining "an accurate comprehension" of what we are doing with our bodies is to pay attention to the sensations in our feet and legs. The first two exercises in this chapter will help you do that. Another help is simply going for a walk, run, or swim *alone*. This can be very centering and grounding. When we are with others, too often the natural social pressures of conversation stop us from turning our attention inward to our body sensations. The benefits of walking, running, or just moving alone come in part from simply being aware of our unprotected moving bodies. Without the "protective shell" of a building or automobile, walkers, runners, swimmers, and bicyclists can feel the weight of the air, temperature, wind on their bodies. Just floating in the experience allows for what has been called an "existential drift," an immediate here-now awareness. This existential drift provides a much-needed break from the stresses of the social world and has a way of putting things into perspective. We are reminded, if only for a little while, of what matters and what does not. Against the backdrop of just being alive and fully in the world, crises take on a different perspective.

Exercise: Swaying and Circling

This is an easy-to-do grounding exercise. It can be done in front of a mirror, but that's not necessary. If you do it with a mirror, start with your eyes closed. Then open them and look in the mirror to see what is actually happening, how you are actually moving in space.

First stand up. If you can't stand, do this sitting on a stool or bed, something that will allow your torso to move freely. Modify the instructions according to what your body can do. If you stand, stand with your feet about shoulder width apart. Flex your knees slightly, and close your eyes. If you feel unsafe or unbalanced with your eyes closed, open them slightly. Now rock forward, leaving your heels on the ground but putting your weight on the balls of your feet. Gently sway back on your heels, keeping your toes on the ground, then forward again and back. Keep doing this slowly. Be aware of your feelings. It's likely you will feel different emotions when you sway backward and then when you lean forward. Going forward, you might feel like you are straining or pushing. Fear often comes up when people lean backwards. It's an automatic response—fear of falling. Both these feelings are emotional reactions to being physically off-balance. Keep your knees slightly flexed to give you more grounding. Try to feel your feet flat on the ground as you're swaying back and forth. Don't get caught up in thoughts and do this exercise just with your head. Feel the movement with your feet and your whole body. And don't forget to breathe. Inhale as you sway forward, and exhale as you go backwards. Repeat this five or six times. Come to a stop in the center.

Keeping your eyes closed, now sway to the right and then to the left, back to the right and then again to the left, moving gently. Again keep your awareness primarily in your feet. Match your breathing to the swaying. Continue swaying for one minute. Feel your feet, your ankles, the weight of your body as it goes back and forth. Don't worry about doing it right or wrong. Come to a stop in the center.

Gently, with your eyes still closed, begin to make a clockwise circle with your torso. Experiment with spreading your feet a little wider to see if you feel more stable. Do what feels right for your body and balance. Again, try to stay out of your head and experience the subtleties of the movement of your body. It may feel like your body is disconnected, head going one way, shoulders another. Moving very much may feel scary or very good. After about one minute, gently come to a stop at center. Now reverse the direction, swaying in a counterclockwise circle. Stop after one minute. Slowly open your eyes. Shake everything out, shaking your arms and legs briefly.

Do you feel more grounded and more settled now than before you began the exercise? Most people do, but you may not. In doing this exercise, some people find the leaning and being off balance very uncomfortable. Did you find yourself gripping the ground with your toes? Those who carry much fear in their bodies find it intensified when they're off-balance, literally or figuratively. Don't judge yourself. Remember, these exercises are not performances. They aren't about getting anything "right." The sole purpose is for you to learn more about getting yourself balanced on the ground beneath you.

This next exercise is practiced at meditation retreats. Walking meditation is a form of meditation training going back centuries. Walking with awareness helps you ground and discharge tension that can build up from long sitting meditations or from any other source of stress. I use it whenever I have trouble sleeping at night. A few minutes of this and a little warm milk seem to do the trick every time.

Exercise: Walking Meditation

The goal of the walking meditation is to keep your focus on the walking and stepping. Begin by walking briskly, saying to yourself "step" each time you put your foot down. Your mind will inevitably wander. Just notice when it does. Gently label the wandering with a descriptive word, such as "thinking" or "remembering." So it might go like this: "Step step step. Step, I should have gotten dog food when I got groceries. Planning. Step, step, step. When am I going to pick the kids up? Planning. Step, step." When you become aware that your mind has gone off-focus, bring it back by repeating the word "step." Walk briskly with focus for two or three minutes. Then slow the walking pace enough to be able to notice both the stepping and the lifting of the foot. Note each part of the action by quietly saying to yourself, "Lift, step, lift, step." Notice what it feels like to be aware of the movements while you are walking. Do this slower walk for another two or three minutes. The final phase of the walking meditation is to lift and step very, very slowly, saying as you move, "Lift, forward, step. Lift, forward, step." The goal is focused awareness with noting. Don't use hard concentration. Just feel the lifting movement, the going forward, the heel going down, and the toe touching. Feel the whole movement. If you find your mind wandering off to "Am I doing this right?" come back to "Step, step, step." Staying focused is difficult, but the settling effect is worth the effort. Don't scold yourself when your mind wanders off, but do gently bring it back. Continue to notice what you feel as you consciously place your feet on the floor. The whole exercise takes six to nine minutes, but you can do it for as long as an hour at a time.

Some people find that when doing the walking meditation exercise they forget to breathe. The process of focusing on the body's sensations may bring up fear and trigger the automatic response of holding the breath. The more you repeat this exercise and all the ones in this book, the better you will know your own response patterns. You will start noticing the times when your breath becomes shallow or rapid and when you are not breathing at all. You might find the slowness of the walking meditation exercise unsettling. When movement is a defense against feelings, slowing down can be very uncomfortable. On the other hand, getting in touch with your movement and the feel of your feet as they contact the ground may be greatly comforting. It is for me. The more movements are reduced to slow motion, the greater the opportunity to be aware of the experience of the moment. Having a few brief moments of not thinking of all the other things that have to be done is a respite. It is a short recess from obligations and gives your mind a rest. For just a few minutes, your mind has to think about only one simple task—walking. It's been said that true healing occurs in those pauses, those brief spaces, when we just are.

When I just can't seem to pull myself together and feel like I'm scattered all over the place, I do this next centering exercise. It's quick and has the effect of consolidating energy. After doing this yoga exercise, I feel like I've successfully rounded up the troops and can again go "Forward! Ho!"

Exercise: Centering Your Energy

Sit on a chair or cross-legged on the floor. Keep your spine erect. Lower your eyelids so they are closed all but one-tenth, leaving them open just a crack. If this is uncomfortable for you, close the lids completely. Raise your eyes under your eyelids so they are focusing on the browpoint. The browpoint is an imaginary spot between your eyebrows and about one inch inside your face.

Now fold your hands in front of your heart. with the palms firmly together in a prayer posture. Exhale and strongly press the palms against each other with your elbows extended out. Apply what seems like about five pounds of pressure. As you inhale, press out with your palms to the sides until the elbows are straight. Keep the wrists bent and the palms facing out as you press away. Now exhale and bring your palms together again in front of your heart. Inhale as you straighten your arms and push out with your palms. Continue this motion, exhaling as you press the palms together and inhaling as you push away. Keep your elbows up. Don't let them droop. Eyes remain closed, with the focus on the browpoint. The spine should be as erect as possible. Continue this movement for seven to eleven minutes. Try to continue the full time even if your arms begin to tire. If you must rest, do so only for one or two breaths and then continue.

At the end of the time, with your eyes still closed, place your left hand over your heart and the right hand over the left. Hold your hands there and breathe deeply for two to three minutes. End the exercise by gently resting your hands in your lap and normalizing your breath. Open your eyes slowly.

Although the exercise is strenuous, the calming and grounding benefits are worth the effort. Use it when you feel scattered and unable to focus or settle down.

The small investment of time in getting grounded in this way is well worth the dividend of being able to harness your energy for whatever tasks follow.

Cara, a client of mine, understands about energy and the need to keep grounded. Her business is computers. When she's not grounded, her computer programs don't work. Cara tells this story: "For two months, I had bugs in a computer program I was working on. It just wouldn't work. Twice it crashed and I lost everything. Then I came to see you, and you said I seemed scattered, that I knew a lot but nothing seemed integrated. That's exactly what was happening with the computer program! I couldn't get one system to integrate with another. You told me to start meditating again. I did, and this is what happened.

"I was sitting on the sofa, just finishing a meditation session. All of a sudden, in my mind I saw this huge black roach crawl out from under the sofa cushion and disappear. It was so real that I immediately opened my eyes to see if I had imagined it or whether there really was a roach crawling beside me on the sofa. No roach. Then I knew something had happened. I went to the computer, turned it on, pulled up the program, and the bugs were gone. The systems integrated and worked together. The problems I had struggled with for two months had vanished like the black roach."

Other electrical problems Cara had been having cleared up equally mysteriously. A food processor she was about to throw out suddenly began to whirl away when she turned it on. Several previous attempts at starting it had been futile. Her hair dryer also had been on the blink. After she began to meditate and got herself grounded, the hair dryer worked fine. Coincidences? That's certainly possible. I prefer to think of them as *co-incidences,* events happening simultaneously that somehow fit together.

Actually, Cara's stories aren't that rare or hard to believe. Each of us has had similar experiences. I know I seem to get all the red lights when I'm rushed and the green ones when I'm flowing internally. When I struggle, things (and objects) around me don't work very well—or at all. The power of our energy shouldn't be underestimated.

One time a client made an appointment to see me together with her husband, which she hadn't wanted to do but did in order to mollify him. She had already decided she wanted out of the marriage and felt this couple's session was only postponing the inevitable. Five minutes before the appointment time, she called me to say their car had stalled on the freeway. The electrical system had shut down. Her husband, an airline pilot, was trying to fix it, but she knew they couldn't make it in time for the appointment. She apologized but felt helpless to do anything about the situation. When I saw her the next week for her individual appointment, I asked how they got the car fixed. "It just started up. We never figured out what happened." I asked her what time the car started. "Right after noon." Their appointment had been scheduled from 11:00 to noon.

Not being grounded affects us socially as well as physically. I have a client, Lynn, who is most vulnerable to losing her sense of being grounded when she's in social situations. Growing up, Lynn always felt she was the ugly duckling of the girls in her family and never fit her mother's image of a girl. While she has resolved most of those issues and has come to accept who she is, the old not-OK feelings rumble when she's in situations where she feels she is being compared with other women. This next exercise is one Lynn uses to help herself stay grounded in her body and not be swept away by all those judgmental and comparing thoughts.

Exercise: Keeping in Touch With Yourself

The exercise is actually quite simple. If you find yourself starting to slip into not-OK inner dialogue in a social situation, touch your middle finger to your thumb tip, making a little circle. Without too much pressure, press the nail of your middle finger to the thumb. The idea is to cause a small sensation that you will be aware of but not pain. You can even do this with your hand in your pocket if you feel self-conscious, but it is a subtle gesture and wouldn't look odd even if someone noticed. Do it with both hands at the same time if you like.

This small amount of unusual pressure will be enough to remind you to come back to yourself, to remember your body, and to stay out of the molasses of comparisons. Repeat as often as necessary. If you notice you are really digging in with your fingernail, take a couple of deep breaths and lighten the pressure. After all, this little technique is to serve as a physical memo, like a string tied around your finger. It's not supposed to be self-inflicted punishment for any imagined failing.

Another valuable way to get grounded is to pay attention to those times when you feel yourself rushing. Rushing doesn't have to do with speed. You can rush sitting still in traffic just as much as racing through the aisles at the grocery store. When we're toppling forward and our minds are ahead of ourselves, we're rushing. At times I find myself rushing while I'm sitting in meditation. These are times, which are all too frequent for many of us, when we have lost our bodies to our thoughts and emotions. Slowing ourselves down and coming back to the present helps us physically as much as mentally. People who chronically feel they are running out of time literally have speeded up biological clocks. The opposite is also true.

There is a teaching in the *Tao Te Ching*, the ancient Chinese book of wisdom, that helps me remember, when I slow down enough to think of it, why rushing is such a mistake. This is the teaching:

> *Rushing into action, you fail.*
> *Trying to grasp things, you lose them.*

Forcing a project to completion,
You ruin what was almost ripe.

This next exercise will help you to slow down internally, even if you have to get things done quickly. I hope it also will help you to avoid ruining some things that are "almost ripe."

Exercise: Stopping the Rushing

When you find yourself rushing, which we all do, stop and take a deep breath. Inhale and exhale slowly. Whether you are standing in a line at the grocery store, waiting for a light to change, or sitting in a doctor's waiting room, pay attention to your body at the moment. Notice which muscles are tight. Your jaw? Your neck and shoulders? The buttocks or stomach? Where in your body are you fighting? As you inhale, try directing your breath into the places in your body where you are fighting against what is happening.

Next, listen to the conversation going on in your head. "My luck! Wouldn't you know I'd get a checkout person who's being trained?! I can't believe how long this is taking!" Be aware of how you are so focused on getting to the next part of your life that you are missing the moment right now. You may think that being stuck in traffic is nothing to miss, but what you are losing out on is the experience of living those minutes, hours, or days peacefully. Instead, you spend them fighting and being angry, impatient, and irritated. Then you have to spend even more of your life recovering from the emotional and physical upset you just added.

We all have plans—many, many plans—about how we want our time to be spent. When you catch yourself rushing, see how you are living in those plans rather than living your life as it unfolds. Settle into the moment. Feel your buttocks on the seat of your car, your feet on the brake or accelerator, and your hands on the steering wheel. Just be where you are. Now look around and see what there is to notice and experience in that moment. Observe the faces of the other drivers or the colors and smells of the food in the grocery store. Open your heart with a little compassion to the others waiting in the doctor's office with you. By doing this regularly, you will discover that your life feels richer and more satisfying and your body carries less pain and stress. Besides, it's a much easier way to live.

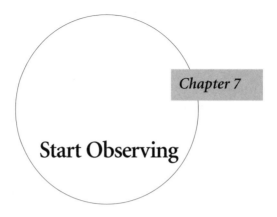

Chapter 7

Start Observing

"The moment you settle down to some fixed view of
things, decay is already setting in."
—*Katsuki Sekida*

It might strike you as odd that observation would
have anything to do with recovering your body. It
does, and very much so. By "observing," I mean
being willing to take the stance of a scientist, gathering
data, and looking at the cold, hard facts of what's happening in your body.

After I had the bodywork treatment for bursitis, I
gradually learned more and more subtle cues about
when my shoulders tighten up. First I noticed that my
right shoulder would tighten when I was angry and
my left when I was frustrated or afraid. They became
like dials on a dashboard that gave me important information as to the state of my "vehicle" as I was driving
down life's highway.

153

I rarely get a headache. When I do, I know it is because I'm holding back feelings so fiercely that my neck and shoulder muscles are constricted into steel bands. They are tightened to the point that the flow of oxygen and blood is sufficiently limited to cause a headache. Sometimes I know what triggers the emotional response I'm fighting; sometimes I don't. I always know, though, that I'm locking in tears, sobs, sorrows, or screams. The holding is so automatic that when it gets to the point of a headache, I can't reason myself out of it. That's when I "get moving." I'll give you an example.

I got a call one night that a friend had died and a memorial service was being held the next day. I hadn't seen Bill or even heard any news about him in several years. That he was dead left me a little stunned, but I got busy reorganizing my schedule so that I could go to the service. I didn't cry then or pay much attention to what I was feeling about his death.

Bill had been a vice-president of a huge insurance company. He was outgoing and well liked. At the Methodist church where the service was to be held, he had served as an elder many years before. When I walked into the big sanctuary of the church, I was completely unprepared for the emptiness. There were fewer than twenty mourners, counting his family and me. I still don't know what happened, why so few people were there to mourn this good-natured man who had extended himself so generously. I sat alone in a pew, listening, watching his ex-wife and children cry quietly. In a few minutes it was over. I spoke the appropriate words to the family and one friend and left—with a headache.

During the afternoon my headache got worse. By the time I got to yoga class at 5:45, my head was throbbing. I started the warm-up exercises, even though it hurt to turn my neck. I kept moving through one asana (posture) after another. My muscles began to loosen, and as they did, the locked-in feelings came gushing out. First I felt waves of sadness. Next came the tears. I rushed to the bathroom and began to sob—great, gut-wrenching sobs. Our yoga classes are usually very quiet and meditative. I know my sobs were heard, but to my immense gratitude, no one stared or said anything when I rejoined the class. Not twenty minutes later, another wave of sorrow and sobs erupted. Back to the bathroom and Kleenex. Finally, my tears stopped. I finished class and left, with almost no headache.

The "scientific discovery" I made from this incident was that my headaches are my damming up sorrow. The concrete wall of rigid neck and shoulder muscles stops my breathing and disconnects my head from my body. My rational self understands this. I know that in part I don't like to cry in front of people because my style of crying is such an event. It's not soft or quiet. I sob. If they ever need extras for a movie at the Wailing Wall in Jerusalem, I'll be hired. When I cry, everyone around knows it. So my body has developed an automatic "face-saving" technique. The obvious problem is that the technique leaves me in pain, emotionally and physically. I have to use breathing and movement to override this well-conditioned response. Overriding it at the moment of emotional upset is not as important to me as understanding and having the data of what my body is doing and why. The more you adopt an observant attitude, the more data you will have. Healer Caroline Myss advises, "If you know what's in your body and where your power centers are, you can close your eyes and see where you lose your power."

You already intuitively know a great deal about where you lose power, even without your eyes closed and even if you don't know what it all means just yet. I encourage my clients to take an observing stance, to attend to what's going on emotionally when they get sick or injured, and to do a kind of personal well-being checkup to see if there might be any correlation between their physical problems and their internal lives. The evidence from the field of psychoneuroim-munology is clear: How we think and how we feel do affect our physical bodies. The exact relationship between your emotions and body awaits your discovery.

My clients have shared with me many of their dis-coveries. Maryjane got arthritis in her hands two weeks after her son died. She had never had it before. She also discovered that she couldn't bend over far enough to pick up the morning newspaper until after she made a decision to divorce. Fred learned that when he was unconsciously dealing with emotional issues related to abuse as a child, his body would start aching. After he addressed the feelings in therapy, the physical pain would be relieved or eliminated. Sue connected the pain in her neck with anger at her husband. I laughingly and truthfully told her, after she made the discovery, that I would sometimes get a pain in the neck after being around her husband, too!

Beth has made a new scientific discovery about her body that both startled and encouraged her in her recovery path. Beth, in her thirties, is an effective accountant. She has had years of therapy to recover from an emotionally abusive upbringing. Even so, her neck and back muscles are in such chronic spasms that she can't stand upright. She began working with a chiropractor and a massage therapist for her back and shoulder pain. Both were helping her. One afternoon as she was lying on the massage table, the massage therapist was working one spot in her left shoulder muscle that had stubbornly resisted all attempts at getting it to release. All of a sudden, Beth saw in her mind a very clear image of a wailing, screaming baby. The baby was her sister at first, and then herself. The image stayed for several seconds. As it faded, she began to sob. She thought she had unleashed some unstoppable force and that she would never be able to quit crying. The tears did stop, though, as they always do sooner or later. Her shoulder felt much better.

The scientific discovery Beth made was that her painful left shoulder muscle holds in the cries she won't let out now and couldn't as a child. "No one wants to be around a whiner," she would say when she felt sadness. Instantly her tears would dry up and her shoulder would tighten. Having made the discovery, Beth doesn't always opt for tears. Usually she doesn't. But she now knows what feelings she is holding in and why. She has recovered that part, those muscles, of her body.

Just as a research scientist never runs out of possibilities of what can be discovered, you can always gather more data about your body. The more you learn, the more you will be recovering your body at both gross and subtle levels. Pay close attention. Keep notes. Don't dismiss any data as unimportant. Believe, at least at first, that everything that happens in your body means something emotionally. Be open and curious about what that might be. Research with the same passion and commitment as a scientist in pursuit of a Nobel Prize. Your own discoveries can be equally rewarding. Your prize will be your own recovered body.

These are some of the areas open for your research and data-gathering: sensations of any kind, posture, breathing, gestures, muscle tension and tightening, blood flow, body temperature, digestion, mannerisms, movements. In short, anything that happens in or with your body could be fertile ground for enlightening discoveries.

To observe like a scientist also means to look objectively at what is happening. I have studied a form of meditation that simply requires observing. It is called Vipassana meditation (see Chapter 14). There are many variations, but the basic process is just observing the breath. Sitting for hours focusing on the breath, you learn to observe dispassionately what is happening to your body, mind, and emotions. One result is learning to allow what is. This objective way of observing is very helpful in coping with painful or frightening emotions or flashbacks. You can learn to note just what is happening instead of judging it with statements such as, "My God, I can't stand it!" The emotions and the pain then pass more easily.

Break down the memory, physical pain, or feelings, as a scientist might, with dispassionate words like "hot, cold, twisting, pressure, burning." Use descriptive kinds of words—*burning, heat, pressure, coolness, squeezing, stretching, contracting, pulsing.* Label what you feel as "fear" instead of "my fear." You will see more of the subtleties of the experience and be less attached to them. The remembering or feeling becomes less upsetting and allows you to see the changes that naturally occur. Eliminate the "my" and "mine" and "this is awful" and "I can't stand it." Taking a more scientific, observant approach to your experiences lessens the emotional and physical suffering. When you begin to analyze the physical pain in detail by noticing the sensations— squeezing, throbbing, pulsing, moving—you are likely to feel less pain, and it often passes more quickly. Even if the pain is chronic and doesn't end, taking an observer's stance seems to help you tolerate it better. It takes some of the suffering out of the pain. Take the "my" and the ownership out of your experience and see if you don't discover that you get through the pain a little easier. Pain and suffering are not the same thing. Suffering is in part our emotional attachment to physical pain. "I can't stand it!" is suffering. "My arm is throbbing" is pain.

Meditation can help you learn to take an observer's stance. Dr. Jon Kabat-Zinn, who directs a stress-management/pain reduction clinic and has taught thousands of patients to meditate, says: "[F]rom a meditative perspective, pain can be a profound experience that you can move into. You don't have to recoil, or run away, or try to suppress it."

He advises that when pain comes up in the body, "See if you can ride the waves of the sensation. As you watch the sensations come and go, very often they will change, and you begin to realize that the pain has a life of its own. You learn how to work with the pain, to befriend it, to listen to it, and in some way to honor it. In the process of doing that, you wind up seeing that it's possible to feel differently about your pain. Sometimes, when you focus on this, the sensations actually go away."

With this kind of objective stance, you can learn to trust all your feelings, that all of them are OK—the pain and the pleasure, hunger and fullness, fear and courage, loneliness and love.

Everyone has the capacity to perceive what is happening in the body with some objectivity. The objectivity may be what gets you through the worst of it.

I know a man named Charlie who has had pain in his gut for most of his adult life. Doctors find no clearly identifiable source for the problem. At times the pain is so bad he throws up and has to go to bed. After Charlie began adopting a scientist's perspective on his pain, he learned a great deal and suffered less. Charlie discovered that the pain began anytime he held in emotions, which he had to do as a child. The pain was also there when he was fatigued or ate too much. He became a specialist on his gut pain. The more he learned, the more encouraged he was. The gut pain isn't gone. It may never be. Charlie suffers much less now, though, and feels much more competent about his body. We are all specialists about our pain, whether we realize it and use that knowledge or not.

Jon Kabat-Zinn had in his clinic a woman with a disregulated hypothalamic condition, which caused her to sweat profusely. While the cause of the condition, perhaps a brain tumor, is still undiagnosed, the woman learned on her own what makes the symptoms better or worse. She attended Kabat-Zinn's clinic, where patients are taught both yoga and meditation. This woman discovered that if she did the yoga without meditating first, she would sweat profusely but when she combined yoga with meditation she did not sweat. Kabat-Zinn concludes, "This is an example of becoming the scientist of one's own mind/body connection."

I have a client with Ménière's disease, a disorder of the inner ear characterized by deafness, dizziness, and a buzzing in the head. While the specialists were running tests and trying out different medications, with no noticeable improvement for her, she was minutely keeping track of the variations in the symptoms and the conditions associated with increased intensity. While she isn't cured, she has learned what to do and what to avoid to minimize the symptoms. She has trained herself to be a careful scientist of her own body and its reaction to psychological, social, and physical factors. You can do that, too.

Exercise: Scientific Observing

This is a quick exercise in observing. Sit or lie down. Notice if the right and left sides of your body are contacting the floor or chair the same way. Probably they are not. Is there a difference in the way one shoulder, hip, foot, or knee contacts the surface? Are your knees different heights from the floor? If you are lying down, notice if your two feet seem to be leaning outward at the same angle? Is one of them pointing straighter toward the ceiling? Notice your face. Can you detect differences in how the right and left sides feel? Can you feel your face at all without putting your hands on it? Can you feel the temperature of your face from within? Can you feel your throat? Is it tight or loose? Is some part of it tight? Notice your shoulders. Are they on the floor or against the back of the chair in the same way? Do they feel sloped forward or pulled back? Is one shoulder higher than the other? Does your chest move as you breathe? Does your rib cage expand with inhalation? Notice your belly, your abdomen. Is it hard or soft? Where? Now be aware of your genitals and your hips. Can you feel them? Perhaps not. Parts of your body may be numb, or you may just feel that a section is just not there. Can you feel your legs? Does the right leg feel different from the left? And the knees? Notice the feet and any tightness in them. Now, very slowly, scan from the top of your head to the bottom of your toes and just see what you notice. Then scan from feet to head. Do this very, very slowly. Just see what you observe, without judging. If you are judging, just observe the judging.

Most people see very little. That is, they see very little of what there is to be seen. Author Annie Dillard says: "It's all a matter of keeping my eyes open. Nature is like one of those line drawings of a tree that are puzzles for children: Can you find hidden in the leaves a duck, a house, a boy, a bucket, a zebra, and a boot? Specialists can find the most incredibly well-hidden things."

Our bodies, part of nature, are like the line-drawing game. We can see so much more if we are willing to look carefully. Becoming a "specialist" who can see incredibly well-hidden things is a matter of practice and intent. You can practice becoming a specialist now with this simple exercise.

Exercise: Seeing the Hidden

Rest your hands, palms down, on a table or on your lap. Notice first how they rest there. Are the fingers close together or spread in a relaxed way? Try letting them soften and relax. Don't struggle or try to force them into some posture. Just notice what happens when you have the intent of letting your hands relax.

Now compare the two hands. Are they very different? Is one larger? Are there differences in color, texture, temperature? Does one seem more masculine or feminine than the other? Turn your hands palm up. What differences do you notice now? Do your hands remind you of someone, perhaps a parent? Note any feelings or judgments that may arise as you make these observations.

Hold your hands out in front of you, palms down. Do they tremble? Is one steadier than the other? Do they seem to want to move in a particular way—into fists, into a prayer posture? Let your hands move for a moment in any way they seem to be drawn.

Now shake your hands and let them relax. Take a deep breath. Turn your attention to only one hand, right or left. Hold it close to your face, just far enough away that your eyes don't blur. What do you see? How does the texture change? What do you see that you didn't see before? Carefully examine each finger, one at a time. Go from the nail down to the web where the fingers join. Look at all sides of each finger. Move your fingers slowly, watching the connections. See how the movements happen. Make a fist slowly and then open your hand one finger at a time. Let the fingers touch and caress each other. Stay aware of as many sensations as you can. Have a child's sense of discovery as you do this. Repeat with the other hand.

Let yourself take at least five to ten minutes to "see the hidden" in your hands. End with an appreciation or prayer of thanks for the miracles we call hands.

This exercise can be used with any part of your body. It is probably best to begin practicing with some body part that you do not associate with pain or shame. Then apply the same exercise to any part of your body that you associate with suffering.

I have given you two exercises in this chapter to help you start observing more carefully what's happening in your body. "Scientific" observing gives you a baseline for measuring changes as you progress in coming alive. The *Seeing the Hidden* exercise will teach you how to look more closely in making observations about your body and its reactions. Both exercises can give you tools that will facilitate your awareness of what your body is needing. The more aware you are, the easier it will be for you to respond to your body's needs. What it needs may be to breathe more deeply, move around, eat, sleep, meditate, have sex, or do one of the exercises in this workbook. Whatever your body requests, fulfilling its needs begins with learning to recognize the requests, and that recognition begins with observation.

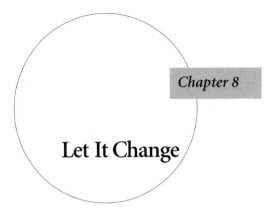

Chapter 8

Let It Change

"The only thing that makes life possible is permanent,
intolerable uncertainty; not knowing what comes next."
—*Ursula K. LeGuin*

Nothing lasts forever. It may feel like forever, but everything does change. The Buddhists talk about change in terms of a concept of impermanence. The Buddha said:

> *This existence of ours is as transient as autumn clouds.*
> *To watch the birth and death of beings is like looking at the movements of a dance.*
> *A lifetime is like a flash of lightning in the sky,*
> *Rushing by, like a torrent down a steep mountain.*

When you are coming back into your body and have been gone for a long time, which most people have, I think it is important to remember that whatever is happening will not be that way forever. It will change. A certain intensity of physical pain will probably be there for only a few minutes. Even with chronic pain or depression, there are variations from moment to moment or hour to hour. So when you have an intense physical pain or a flashback of traumatic memories, if you can remind yourself that this is going to pass, the fear will lessen. It will end. Not ignoring the experience but allowing it to happen with awareness lets you learn from the experience. It is less frightening if you know it will end. Here the concept of impermanence, that everything changes, can be of great comfort. Tibetan master Sogyal Rinpoche suggests that "impermanence is like some of the people we meet in life—difficult and disturbing at first, but on deeper acquaintance far friendlier and less unnerving than we could have imagined." Being mindful of impermanence allows you to ride with the experience, to stay with it. This is Annie Dillard's advice: "Not only does something come if you wait, but it pours over you like a waterfall, like a tidal wave. You wait in all naturalness without expectation or hope, emptied, translucent, and that which comes rocks and topples you; it will shear, loose, launch, winnow, grind." And you will be healing while you allow the changing to happen.

I am not a big fan of scary rides, like roller-coasters. It is not my idea of fun. I like to climb mountains with my husband, Blair, to go to the big peaks. When I'm climbing, most of the time I have control of where my feet are going. On a roller-coaster, I am definitely not driving, and once I buy my ticket and get on the ride, I give up control. Recovering the body is at times like riding the roller-coaster. If you can try not to fight what happens by remembering that at some point the ride will stop, the whole process will flow more easily.

Arthur hits pillows and screams in the night. It started after he had a stroke. That's when Arthur first started coming alive. He was sixty years old then. Until that time, he was a workaholic, albeit a very successful one. Valium and other medications helped him to control his "nervous stomach" for several decades. Even with those medications, Arthur drank and raged.

He didn't know it at the time, but Arthur was terrified. He had been afraid since he was a baby, afraid no one loved him. I'm not sure anyone really did. He married, had kids, worked hard, built a big, solid manufacturing company. Then he had the stroke. The doctors took him off all the medications, and his feelings came to the surface in torrents. The anxiety he experienced was so intense he had to be hospitalized. For months afterwards, he couldn't bear to be alone. He panicked and raged if his wife had to go out of town or even stay late at a meeting.

"All those feelings have been waiting to come out for decades," I told him. "Let go and quit fighting them." He protested that he felt so overwhelmed by the feelings that he was afraid for them to start. "They will stop, sooner or later. Just let them come," I tried to reassure him. Chaos is opportunity. Arthur's chaos was the opportunity for him to learn to feel again.

He did let the feelings come. When unconscious terror would jolt Arthur upright in bed from his sleep, he would march to the utility room, grabbing sofa pillows on the way. With the door shut, he would get on his knees and begin pounding the pillows and screaming. Sometimes only wordless sounds came out. Sometimes gut-wrenching sobs followed the screams. One night he heard himself scream, "Don't leave me! Please love me! I hate you!" Then he heard "I hate me!" and sobbed.

The words he bellowed stunned Arthur. For the first time, he understood how his fear was connected to his self-hatred. What mattered as much as his understanding and insight, though, was that he was releasing long-pent-up rage and cries for help and love that had been stifled for six decades.

The trips to the utility room were nightly at first. Sometimes he was there for hours. After two years of his faithfully being with his body, the nocturnal trips are infrequent. The release takes less time. Arthur now finds himself rocking and clutching a pillow more than yelling. He feels his loneliness, his unlovableness, and stays with those feelings. When he goes back to bed, he sleeps more easily.

Resisting what is happening can impede recovery and prolong suffering. You can resist the flow of healing by declaring "I am not going to let this happen, and it is not coming. I am just not going to do this!" But you will delay your recovery and pay a price. If you willfully stop what your body and unconscious are trying to release, the internal struggle persists. Healing simply takes longer.

I have a client, Jane, who was determined not to feel or show vulnerability. She had learned as a child that doing so would only bring more shaming and blaming, never any comfort. When her tears threaten to spill out, this stoic woman makes a fist and slams it against whatever surface is closest. Jane is determined to beat her pain back inside. Automatically, her jaws tighten and thrust forward. Her neck and shoulder muscles become rigid. Not surprisingly, she suffers from intense depression and chronic physical pain. Sogyal Rinpoche wisely says: "We are terrified of letting go, terrified, in fact, of living at all, since learning to live is learning to let go. And this is the tragedy and the irony of our struggle to hold on: Not only is it impossible, but it brings the very pain we are seeking to avoid."

You may have been uncertain about buying a ticket for this recovery ride, or any ride in life, for that matter, but once you are on it and strapped in, you might as well see what it's like. Learning to think like a scientist helps make the ride less overwhelming. "Now we are going up. Now down. Now this is happening. Now that." That's what I mean by "let it change." Stay with it and let it change, because it will.

My experience in meditating is that it is very common to have a muscle start hurting when I sit unmoving for an hour. Part of the discipline of meditating is that you do not move during a sitting. The protocol is not to scratch your nose or anything else, to resist those impulses. The reason for not moving is in part to learn directly the experience of impermanence. What you learn is that even if you do not move, the muscles stop hurting sooner or later anyway. The itch passes. The problem is gone or changed. But if you scratch or wiggle or get up, you believe that you are the one that has to solve all problems, that it is only because you did something that the pain stopped. Not doing something can be as effective as taking action and is often more so.

I once was in a body therapy workshop with other therapists, many of whom had been physically or sexually abused. They knew that the two days of exercises we were about to embark on were designed to bring up emotions and memories, which they did. At the beginning of the workshop, the instructors asked each person to say one word that would best describe what he or she was feeling at that moment. Common responses were "dread" and "fear." When my turn came, I said "excited." Some of the participants looked at me as if to say, "This lady doesn't know what she's doing. She just doesn't know what she's in for!" I did know. After twenty years of body therapy, I now welcome whatever is going to come up. For me, it is like vomiting up poisonous food. I know I am going to feel so much better afterwards that I am open to the experience. I do indeed feel excited and enthusiastic about whatever comes, even the suffering. I know from experience the prizes that are connected to the release: physical and emotional peace, sometimes even improvement from an illness, like a cold or, infection. I am willing to pay the price for those prizes. Our bodies and psyches are always trying to heal themselves. If we just allow it and don't fight it, unimaginable gifts await us.

One of the most direct ways of learning to "let it change" is to realize how much change we allow our bodies to experience every day. The living body is always changing. All experience alters the body in some way. Every experience produces many kinds of changes: electrical, chemical, glandular, muscular. We are unconscious of most of these fluctuations. Maybe we are aware of the more gross changes, but most of the subtle ones escape our notice.

Here is an exercise in noticing the normal gross as well as subtle changes in your body. Try it once. If you find it comforting, do it for a few minutes every day for a week or longer. Then let it go for a while. If you find yourself resisting what is happening in your body, you can always go back to this exercise.

Exercise: Seeing the Body Change

Reflect for a moment on all the physical changes that you take for granted each day. You wake up with some sleepiness, gradually become more alert as you have a cup of coffee, shower, do exercises, meditate, or whatever you do to get going. At different times in the day, you find your alertness alters. Mid-morning or mid-afternoon drowsiness is common. As your normal bedtime approaches, you find yourself sleepier and ready to recline or go on to sleep.

Similar changes take place with hunger. People vary in when they experience hunger, but, unless we are ill, we do get hungry. The body sends out signals that it needs food. We eat, and the experience of hunger changes. For most people, this cycle repeats itself several times in a twenty-four-hour period. Elimination is another bodily function that reflects many changes in the course of a day. We experience the need to go to the bathroom, go, and feel relief. The feeling of urgency changes.

Body temperature fluctuates all through the day and night. Some of the fluctuation or change is due to internal regulation. Temperature shifts because of environmental changes, cooler or warmer air in the room, going outside, exercising. Even which nostril we breathe through more shifts every two hours or so. This, like many other body changes, is something most people do not notice consciously.

After taking a few moments to realize how you experience continuous changes in your body, take one period, ten to fifteen minutes, to consciously note and record every body change, however subtle, that happens. What muscles tighten or loosen during that period? What itches that was not itching a few moments before? When does hunger begin or end? Does some ache start, cease, intensify or lessen? Do you get hotter or cooler? Do you need to go to the bathroom? Does the need intensify during the observation period? What happens after you go?

Being aware of the remarkable process of change and adjustment that is occurring at all times in the body can give you greater confidence that your own pain will change if you allow it to do so. The body is always striving for balance and wholeness. Seeing that reality through this brief observation can give you the courage not to stop the process.

Much of what drives addictive and habitual behaviors is the unwillingness and inability to stay with a feeling, urge, or craving long enough for it to change. We feel sad or needy and act (with drugs, sex, spending, work, eating) before we have a chance to see what might happen to those feelings if we did nothing. Doing nothing might be worse, for a while, or it might be better. Either way, something will change. This little exercise is to serve as a practice in doing nothing when you feel an intense urgency to act on a craving or impulse.

Exercise: Seeing into the Future/Moving Past Now

The next time you find yourself really wanting something—anything—stop! Just stop and turn your attention inward for one minute. Notice what is happening in your body. Are your hands starting to tremble? Is your breath getting more rapid? Your body is most probably tensing somewhere. Where? Are you salivating? Are your eyes tearing up? Are sexual feelings starting or intensifying?

Listen to the dialogue in your head. "I've got to have that! It/she/he is exactly what I've been looking for! I've got to get it now or it will be gone!" Just listen. Listen and feel what is happening in your body.

It's not wrong to get excited about something. It's great. Life would be a big bore if we never let ourselves get excited about what we want. The passion would be missing. The problem comes when our passions become automatic and block authentic living.

Stop yourself from acting just long enough to fully recognize what is happening in your body and in your mind at the moment of craving and desiring. Take careful note. You can still have it. Just pause long enough to see what is happening.

If you made it this far, push yourself a little farther. Tolerate your desiring just a bit longer without acting. Imagine now that it is one month from this moment. One month from now, do you still want that dessert, drink, dress, man/woman? Go on into the future. It's six months from this moment. What has happened to your craving? Do you still passionately want that new car, business deal, cocaine? Observe what's happening in your body. Keep going. All this need only take a few minutes. A year from now? Five years? Now stop. Come back to this moment. What do you feel in your body? In your emotions? Take three deep breaths. Now imagine breathing in the warm, healing Golden Light. Breathe it into your chest, your solar plexus, an energy center. Breathe in the Golden Light for one or two minutes. Breathe into your pure center. Now make your choice about how you are going to act. However you decide to respond to your craving, you do so more consciously and with the knowledge that it is indeed a choice you are making. Whether you take what you long for or let go, you will now act with more awareness.

You may be surprised or even disappointed to discover how quickly your passion or craving fades. I heard a story once about a man who wanted more and more of the best. Don't we all know that guy? He worked hard and could afford to buy the best of everything. One day he went to pick up his new sports car. He had waited months for it to arrive. It cost more than most people's houses and was beautiful. He climbed into the leather seats, put his hands on the precisely engineered steering wheel, glanced with delight at the glittering array of gauges and dials, took a deep drag of the new car smell, started the engine, pulled out onto the street, and drove away in bliss. Bliss lasted six blocks. He was terrified when he realized that his multi-thousand-dollar fix lasted less than fifteen minutes. Nothing had changed about the car. The only change was in him.

Most of us do better than that in making our passions last longer. But the same thing happens to everyone all the time. Joy fades. Anger fades. Everything changes. The more we insist that something or someone keep us up or high, the more quickly we will be let down. Genuine, lasting highs come only from accepting every moment of the changes—the highs and the lows. Looking into the future gives you a small opportunity to anticipate the changes and to act with that knowledge. You may still choose to get what you initially desired, but you are less likely to be surprised that the fix doesn't last. No fix lasts. It's not supposed to, and it can't.

This *Getting Dizzy* exercise is to give you a controlled taste of how you can be spinning out of control and your body will right itself if you give it the chance. It's also fun. After all, it has probably been a good, long time since you spun around just for the fun of it. A word of caution: If you have high blood pressure or vertigo, best to skip this exercise. Otherwise, let'er rip!

Exercise: Getting Dizzy

Stand in the middle of a room, where you can swing your arms without hitting anything or hurting yourself. Raise your arms out to the side. Keep your eyes open. Now start spinning. Spin until you are good and dizzy. (It takes only a few seconds.) Stop gently.

Carefully sit or lie down. Close your eyes. Feel the spinning. Feel your disorientation. Notice any feelings. Is it fun? Scary? Confusing? Notice how the dizziness begins to fade. It probably will fade within seconds. If you continue to feel dizzy, open your eyes and look at the ceiling or straight ahead. Stay resting until you feel steady again.

The point of this exercise is to enable you to experience very immediately how your body can steady you when you are off-balance without your doing anything. It has a built-in balancing system, many of them, actually. The *Getting Dizzy* exercise can help you to trust those systems a little more, to learn to believe that if you can allow the process of change to continue, your experience will change.

Children like to spin themselves, to get dizzy. No one has to teach them or tell them it's a good thing to do. They just do it for the fun of it. I believe we all need to be dizzy and out of control at times, by choice or not. I like it better, of course, when I can have some control over my being out of control. But that choice is not always available. Flashbacks don't usually come by choice. Neither do traumatic memories. Like birth and death, they come when they come. Since dizziness in life is inevitable, my advice is to get used to it and to learn to trust that dizziness will be followed by steadiness followed by dizziness followed by steadiness. ... Let go of trying to hold onto what has to change, and respect the wisdom of changing. *We* are the ones who keep ourselves dizzy by continuing to spin and spin. When we stop, calmness, stillness, and clarity will come again. They always do. Trust that. Someone once said, "There's a rhythm to God. It's agony and ecstasy." Do the *Getting Dizzy* exercise until you do trust the natural process. Ride the carnival rides until you believe, without a doubt, that the wild ride will end and you'll walk on solid ground again.

Learning to let our bodies naturally change is a lesson we must practice all our lives. Once, my husband and I were attending a professional meeting in San Francisco. I caught a cold a couple of days after we got there. Two days later, my cold was turning into a sinus infection. I began to get scared. Historically, when I get a sinus infection, it turns into bronchitis. With bronchitis, I cough all night and I can't breathe well. During the night, I realized I was getting really sick. I lay propped up in the big hotel king-size bed next to Blair, trying very hard not to cough and wake him again, as I had done every few minutes since we had turned out the lights. I could feel my lungs start to tighten. I knew the infection was spreading and my panic along with it. I remembered all those nights as a child when I had lain next to my mother, propped up on the pillows, trying not to wheeze so that I wouldn't awaken and alarm her. I felt very small and very alone that night in San Francisco.

I got up out of the bed and went into the bathroom. I began to cough, trying to clear my throat and the airways clogged with mucous. Suddenly tears began to come. I leaned on my elbows, my head over the sink. Spasms of coughing exploded out of me, followed by sobs—huge, breathless sobs. My entire body shook with fear. Blair came in, understandably concerned. I couldn't manage any word of explanation. I just clung to him and felt the stalking terror of death I had felt as a child. More choking coughs, more sobbing, more terror wracking what felt like the body of a child, five or six years old, maybe younger. It seemed the ordeal would never stop, but I didn't resist. Twenty minutes, and it was over.

The next morning my sinus infection had cleared up considerably. I wasn't completely well, but I was much healed. I never did get bronchitis. I took antibiotics a few days later to clear up the sinus infection. I'm not sure what triggered that eruption of terror. Certainly getting sick was a big part of it. Maybe it was being in a strange bed, as I was so often when I became ill as a child. The fact that I had been writing about my childhood asthma the day before for this book was probably a contributing element. Regardless of why it happened, I knew my job was to "let it change," to let the feelings and body-held pain follow their own course.

The unconscious has a path it follows as certain ly as a river knows to flow to the ocean. To build a dam across the natural path of the flow always has consequences, some potentially destructive. My unconscious path to healing that night had to do with sobbing, coughing, and being terrified. I'm grateful I wasn't alone, but I would have tried to go through it even if I had been. The wisdom of the unconscious as manifested in the body is a precious gift, one I'm not willing to push away.

Is that the last of my fear connected to my asthma? Will it happen again the next time I get bronchitis? I have no idea and actually no preference one way or the other. If there is more pain buried in my body, in my lungs or anywhere else, I'll meet it when it shows up, like someone from the past that we encounter unexpectedly. Those encounters can be transformative. Sometimes they put an end to some unfinished business. Other times they open new possibilities or doors to new awareness. Whatever I meet in recovering my body, whenever, wherever, however, I plan to continue to see what happens and let my body change as it will.

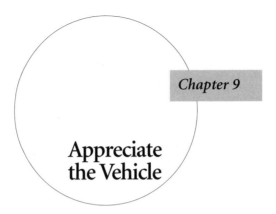

Chapter 9

Appreciate the Vehicle

"And all must love the human form,
    in heathen turk or jew;
Where Mercy, Love and Pity dwell
There God is dwelling too."
                    —*William Blake*

M
any religious teachings talk about the body's being the temple of the soul or the clay vessel that carries life. But even the religious can fail to honor the glory of the physical body. Gabrielle Roth tells this story:

"I ran into a rabbi in a shopping mall. We got to talking and I asked, 'Do Jews hate their bodies as much as Catholics?' He started to laugh in mock shock, but then gave me a more quizzical look. It seemed I'd hit on something close to him. He told me that he'd just buried his father, who was also a rabbi. He'd asked his father on his deathbed, 'What was

the most important thing in your life? The *Torah?*'
And the old man had answered, 'My body.'

"'I was stunned,' his son now told me. He stared
past me in awkward silence and finally said, 'I always
thought my body was just a vehicle for my mind; feed it,
clothe it, send it to Harvard.'"

Pain and illness in our bodies can make us forget to
be appreciative of this vehicle that carries soul and life
around. If your life has been one of pain, you may be
angry that this thing called a body keeps you here on
earth, but hating your body won't get you out of it any
faster and definitely is not a step to recovering it.
Appreciating it, regardless of its shape, size, or condition
is a positive step. Poet, scholar, and mystic Andrew
Harvey declares, "What is needed is for the body to be
blessed. Why? Because we're in it. Why would we be
here if we weren't meant to love and celebrate our bodies, and to ennoble and irradiate the joys of the body
with the wisdom of the soul, and to find out that sexuality can be the physical grammar of the lovemaking of
the soul? That's what we're here to find out."

I remember standing nude in front of the full-
length mirror. Turning sideways and sucking in my
belly, I thought, "Just a little more, and it will be just
right." The reflection I saw was of a ninty-eight-pound,
5'5" tall, twenty-two-year-old woman. That body had
nothing to do with me. It was an object. My goal was to
make it "right," to fit the image of the ideal body in
vogue at the time. The time was mini-skirts and the

model Twiggy (who weighed eighty-nine pounds and was 5'7"). The ideal woman's body shape was that of an adolescent boy. No breasts, no hips. Straight. I was nearly there.

I feel sadness even now thinking of the lack of compassion I showed for that body. Ignoring hunger pangs, wearing binding clothes that cut off circulation, I never thought about whether I needed food, exercise, or rest. Strong coffee and even diet pills were my weapons against fatigue.

It is no surprise that my body fought back in response to such abusive treatment. I was constipated; had excruciating menstrual pains; caught the flu often; had sinus infections, chronic allergies, aching neck, and shoulder pain; and I drank a lot. What else could I expect? My body had no life in it. It was telling me in every way possible that I was doing things all wrong, but I couldn't begin to see a connection. Many of my clients have done great harm to their bodies, and they, like me as a twenty-two-year-old, see little connection between what they are doing and the health of their bodies.

Hannah is a beautiful young woman. She dresses with flair and has bright eyes and an easy, infectious laugh. Men and women turn to stare—and smile—when they see Hannah. Despite being beautiful, Hannah was ruthlessly addicted to men who abused her and were desperate to be with her. She was sexually abused by her father, and her mother tried to kill her when she was two.

A few months after I met Hannah, she announced to me that she would be missing the next week's appointment. "I'm going to get a boob job," she laughed gaily. "I think my clothes will hang better on me if I have larger breasts. I've wanted to do it for some time, so now I'm going to."

My protests were futile. I urged her to wait a few months. I told her I thought she would feel different about her body in the future, that she wouldn't want the surgery then. But her mind was set. Hannah had the surgery. She suffered much pain and had complications. That was four years ago. Now she wonders about the safety of the implants and what she should do, whether or not to have them removed or changed. It was all so unnecessary.

If Hannah had been able to appreciate the healthy body that carries her soul, had she been able to see the function instead of the form, she would not have had to submit to mutilation and pain. Now her body looks "perfect," like some ideal, and it will remember always the unnecessary pain she subjected it to.

Sam, in contrast, sees his body as literally a pain in the neck. He doesn't think about his body unless he's hungry, horny, or hurt. Lately, he has been hurting a great deal. Sam sees absolutely no connection between the terrible neck and back pain he suffers and the rage he is holding back. How he "injured" his neck is a mystery to him, and he steadfastly refuses to hear my suggestions that his physical and emotional pain are connected. He may be catching on, though. He reported to me that after a fight with his wife, his back seared with pain. Even so, Sam is a very long way from "appreciating the vehicle," from being able to thank his body for being an astute teacher that lets him know when he is out of balance emotionally. I hope he catches on soon. His suffering is crippling.

I'm not sure people know how to think about the body and the spirit it houses. Jesuit priest and poet George McCauley ponders the ambivalence in his poem "On the Mend":

> *Some say the body holds*
> *the spirit up like*
> *a corset, is its eyes and*
> *ears, displays its moods,*
> *points it to its prey,*
> *retrieves what the spirit*
> *desires, and gets a pittance*
> *in return—in fact is*
> *ridiculed because the spirit*
> *thinks it's hot stuff,*
> *wants everything all*
> *at once and cannot stand*
> *the body's ponderous delay.*
> *But others say the spirit*
> *is the body's friend, takes*
> *it everywhere, dresses it*
> *up, introduces it around,*

makes a name for it,
conceals its unseemly
parts, abides its
nervous schedules, gets it
to laugh, keeps the noise
down while the body sleeps.

Maybe most of us believe both things at one moment or another.

Clarissa Pinkola Estés talks about the price a woman or man pays by falling prey to beliefs about how a body "should" look or be. She says angst about the body robs a person of a large share of creative life and attention to other things. It has been her observation that "many people treat their bodies as if the body is a slave, or perhaps they even treat it well but demand it follow their wishes and whims as though it were a slave nonetheless." More important, she declares, "is not what shape, what size, what color, what age, but does it feel, does it work as it is meant to, can we respond, do we feel a range, a spectrum of feelings? Is it afraid, paralyzed by fears, anesthetized by old trauma, or does it have its own music, is it listening, … is it looking with its many ways of seeing?" She urges us to remember that the body is "a being in its own right, one who loves us, depends on us, one to whom we are sometimes mother, and who sometimes is mother to us."

Our bodies are the best mothers we can ever hope to

have. My body knows when I am hungry, thirsty, sleepy, sick, needing to play, run, or have sex. It knows what I am feeling as soon as I feel it. It is always right about whether I need warmer clothes or when my shoes pinch. But like a preoccupied child or a rebellious teenager, I sometimes ignore this wise mother. "Not now. I don't want to! Later!" Those are our responses to the Body Mother who truly does know best. Learning to appreciate the vehicle is learning to have more respect for the wisdom of that "mother," no matter what her shape.

Just think of how amazing our infant body was. Chuang-tzu, in commenting on the fifty-fifth teaching in the *Tao Te Ching,* says this: "The infant cries all day long without straining its throat. It clenches its fists all day long without cramping its hand. It stares all day long without weakening its eyes. Free from all worries, unaware of itself, it acts without thinking, doesn't know why things happen, doesn't need to know. This mode of being in our body, our original home, at one with the whole world, is still present in us." We just have to be willing to go home again.

Appreciating the vehicle also means appreciating the scar tissue that has grown over our wounds. The psychic wounds we suffer in childhood can give us the strength we need to endure adversity. Scar tissue is the strongest tissue in the body. It may look deformed or unattractive, but it's tough. Severe emotional wounds that cut us deeply can make for toughness that contributes to our survival. People who anticipate all the bad things that can happen to them in surgery actually recover better than those who don't think about the problems and pain that might result from the operation. Scaring yourself a little helps you to build coping strategies and defenses. When you have been abused or shamed as a child, those early wounds forced you to grow psychic scar tissue that protects you to this day. If that psychic scar tissue is kept supple, stretched, and soft, it need not bind you in a crippling manner.

Monica Seles couldn't look at her scar tissue. The world's top-ranked tennis star was stabbed in the back by a deranged man in Hamburg, Germany, on April 30, 1993, as she sat in a chair on the court during a tennis match. Months after the assault, she said, "I didn't look at the injury, I still can't. I've never looked in the back. … It's not something that I want to do. It just reminds me too much of what happened." I think that's a big mistake. We have to look, or the pain stays with us. At the time she was interviewed, Monica Seles had not swung a tennis racket since the day of the attack. She was left with chronic nightmares, in which she saw a man with a red face standing just behind her with a raised knife. He had already stabbed her once and is about to do it again. I hope some day she will be able to look at that scar and go through the terror and out the other side. That's what we all have to do with our wounds and scars if we're not to be crippled by them.

I once overheard a woman explaining about burled wood. She pointed to a tree across the park. Its trunk was covered with tumor-like growths. Burls, she explained, happen when lightning strikes or diseases damage the tree. On the outside, the tree looks deformed. But the damaged wood has intricate swirling patterns that can be used to make beautiful veneers, bowls, table tops, and sculptures. The unique beauty of the wood comes from the wounding. The woman said to her friend, "I think that we're all like that tree. We've all been damaged, but beauty comes out of our hurts." She's so right. Our own patterns of beauty come from our particular woundings and make possible a creation that could come only from us.

Fred was missing the end of his right ring finger. He cut it off with a jigsaw in shop class forty years ago. That missing joint had come to symbolize for Fred all of his shame about so many things he lacked, love above all. He kept his hand somewhat hidden, unconsciously trying to hide his flaws, external and internal. One day I took his wounded hand and asked him to tell me the story of what happened. His buried sorrow was so intense that tears welled up in *my* eyes, not his. All I could say as I gently stroked the damaged finger was, "I'm so sorry that happened to you." No one had ever said that to Fred when he was growing up, about his finger or any other wounding. Fred said nothing in reply. Later he told me that he thought I was making fun of him. But he let the words stay in his heart and began to say them to himself. "I'm so sorry this happened to me." Slowly he allowed a compassion for his body and all it had endured. Eventually he was able to share his wounds with others and receive their compassion in return. He learned to accept kindness and told me years later the lesson he had learned: "When someone said something good to me, you taught me to inhale and feel it and say 'Thank you.'"

Lütfiye, my meditation teacher, once said, "Rita, if we were on a sinking ship, I would want to be standing next to you." What she meant was that I am very good at taking action in a crisis. I don't freeze. The action I take may not be the most well thought-out, but I do something. That's some of my scar tissue. My mother wasn't the kind who tolerated helplessness or weakness. You straightened your shoulders, sucked in your gut, and went on. Her tough thinking and planning, and later my own, shielded me from feeling overwhelmed as a child. It was my shelter during life's invariable tidal waves. It's still a struggle for me to let someone, or even myself, know when I'm feeling helpless. That psychic scar tissue isn't completely flexible and probably never will be. But the gift of the scar tissue is an absolute conviction that I can take care of myself, and I'm grateful for that. Work to appreciate the gift in your own psychic scar tissue, no matter how ugly the wound.

Psychic scar tissue also may produce spiritual scar tissue, which is the best kind of all. Kids who learned to turn to God in their suffering, and many do, build a faith that is really tough. They end up with a spiritual knowledge of God that holds them fast no matter how bad the emotional or physical storm raging in the family around them. Spiritual scar tissue can grow at any time in our lives, if we allow it.

Sarah was enraged at God. "Where was He when all those atrocities were being committed on me?" She was right to rage and wrestle with her God until she came up with some answers. For her, the answer came in knowing that God had been in there with her in the suffering and abuse, in her pain, beside her and inside her. That's Sarah's spiritual scar tissue.

Exercise: Learning to Appreciate

This exercise is designed to help you regain some appreciation for your body. Allow five to ten minutes. Sit or stand in front of a full-length mirror. Begin by just witnessing what you are thinking and feeling when you do this. What you may first notice is judgment: Part is too fat or too skinny or even ugly. Be aware of the judgments. Then look into your own eyes. Just look. See what you see. Ask yourself, "Have I changed since I was a child, or am I the same? Are those the same eyes?" Really look. You may have to look at childhood pictures to see if your eyes are the same eyes you had as a child. Are there any differences between the person you see in the mirror and the person you feel yourself to be? You might be quite surprised by what you see when you look objectively. You have an image of yourself as a cheerful person, and yet you see someone who looks very sad. What do you like or dislike about what you see? Notice both what you like and what you do not.

Now stop observing and close your eyes for a few seconds. Take a deep and relaxing breath and let go of your judgments. With your eyes closed, think of a self-loving affirmation. Remind yourself that what you saw in the mirror is a soul that was created by God, and that you are here for some important purpose. To demean that soul is to demean all souls. Be open to the possibility of seeing this person, this soul, you see in the mirror in a new and different way. End with the Golden Light imaging. With each inhalation, see or feel a Golden Light flowing into that part of you that remains pure. Let it fill your body with loving, healing energy. The Light is flowing into the pure part of you, the part that will always remain perfect, undefiled, age-less, whole. As the Light touches and penetrates you, allow it to cleanse and purify all your wounds, pain, suffering, destructive emotions, and shame. Let yourself be dissolved into the Light, even if only for a moment. Rest in this renewing, restoring Light. As the Presence fades, express your "thank you" for the body you have, knowing it has served you honorably and is now a little different, a little healed.

Open your eyes slowly. Look in the mirror. Notice what, if anything, looks different from a few minutes before. Doing this exercise on a regular basis is very powerful. Try to do it at least once a month. If you know you carry shame about your body, do it weekly for six weeks, and then once a month. Even if it's very hard at first, stick with it. It will help.

Sometimes it helps us to appreciate the body more by realizing how many different "vehicles" we have actually traveled in and how each has served us in ways that were appropriate to the changing stages of our lives. The *Different Bodies* exercise will help you to look back at your different bodies.

Exercise: Different Bodies

This exercise takes some preliminary organization. Gather photos of yourself, as many as are available or can be obtained, from every age of your life: newborn or baby, toddler, as a little child, older childhood, teen years, up to the most recent photos you have of yourself. Include full-length photos if you have them.

Set aside a time when you are not likely to be disturbed for a half-hour or longer. Spread the photos out in front of you in chronological order—youngest to present day. Take a few minutes just to see the evolution of your own body. See how many different bodies you have obviously had. Try to remember as much as you can of what it felt like to be in each of those bodies that you see before you.

Slowly, picture by picture, thank each body for carrying you through that period of your life. Appreciate the uniqueness of each body you had and how it was exactly suited to the life tasks facing you at the time. Acknowledge the soft flexibility of your baby body, the growing strength of the legs of your toddler body, the awkwardness or beauty of your adolescent body, the maturity or fertility of your adult body. When you remember or see problems in any of these bodies— pain, illness, deformity, obesity, look with compassion on the suffering that body carried on your behalf. Give thanks for all it did and is doing to help you cope and survive. Put all the pictures together and embrace them, as you would hold a beloved infant, to your heart. Love the vehicles that have brought you so far and through so much. End with the Golden Light imaging from the previous exercise.

This exercise may bring up intense feelings and critical judgments. If it is too much for you right now, set it aside and try again later, perhaps in a few days, weeks, or months. Keep doing the exercise until it is not only easy but enjoyable.

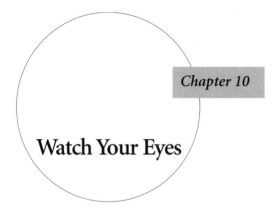

Chapter 10

Watch Your Eyes

"In our minds there is an awareness of perfection
  and when we look with our eyes we see it."
  —*Agnes Martin*

Seeing is about looking. How we look reflects how we see life and how we feel. Christ said, "The eye is the lamp of the body. So if your eye is clear, your whole body is luminous; but if your eye isn't clear, your whole body is dark."

I come from a long line of Blemish players. A Blemish player is someone who has mastered the art of seeing a flaw in everything. The new art exhibit isn't as skillfully presented as the one the museum had two months ago. The fajitas at the Mexican restaurant aren't as good as they were before the restaurant moved to its new location. The azaleas this year weren't anything compared to three years ago. Blemish players see what is wrong with life, not what's right. It's a guaranteed system for feeling disappointed. The soul and body are deprived of the experience of joy and delight that comes from unconditional acceptance of what is. We cheat ourselves by how we see.

I once had a teacher who amazed me in her indefatigable ability to find something good in everything that happened. She wasn't a Pollyanna who pretended nothing was bad. But she looked with eyes that saw what was right, while I looked with eyes trained to see what was wrong. It took me years to change how I see. Now it's as automatic for me to see with optimistic, appreciative eyes as it used to be to see with critical, rejecting eyes.

There's no real exercise in this section to teach you to relinquish Blemish playing. But if you are interested in giving up the game of taking the "Ain't It Awful" view of your life and in looking through rosier glasses, give some consideration to playing "Ain't It Wonderful" instead. It's no harder and much more fun. Your body will appreciate it, too. How you look literally affects how you feel emotionally and physically. The reverse is also true. What is happening in you emotionally affects how you see.

A chronic, vigilant, on-guard attitude toward life is

mirrored in tension in the eyes. The muscles are tense and strained. Nearsightedness can be one result. With nearsightedness, you can see what is up close, within your reach or control. What's hard to see are those things in the distance, the unknown, the uncontrollable.

Not everyone wants to see clearly. My ophthalmologist told me that. Measurements for vision correction are always made both objectively and subjectively. That's why they ask us, "Which makes it better? This? Or this?" Seeing with hard, clear edges makes some people uncomfortable. "Some like it a little blurry," my ophthalmologist mused. Seeing life clearly takes getting used to. Don't rush any changes in how you see, literally or metaphorically. Changing how you see the world takes time. It happens anyway, but we can nudge it along in a direction of our choice.

I am nearsighted and have been for thirty years, the same amount of nearsighted all that time. When I was a senior in high school, we were all gathered in the auditorium for school assembly. I realized I couldn't see very clearly what was going on up on the stage. It was an assembly awarding certificates to National Merit Scholars. I wasn't one, although I was a conscientious and good student. I believe the future got blurry for me then and stayed that way.

Steven Vazquez, a psychotherapist and a masterful healer with his hands, says that eye problems relate to three emotional issues: 1) holding back tears and being unwilling to cry when your body needs to cry; 2) not wanting to see something that is difficult to face; or 3) problems with "I," as in identity—"Who am I?" All three of those issues applied to me in the school auditorium that afternoon. I was sorely disappointed and felt like crying, I'm sure, but I wasn't willing to face my disappointment in myself. As a high school senior, I was definitely struggling with the existential issue of "Who am I?" My eyes didn't become nearsighted on that one afternoon, but I believe the tension and vigilant attitude with which I viewed life reached a certain critical threshold that day, and the distance looked fuzzy from then on … until recently, anyway.

In my persistent quest to see what my body can teach me, I sought out "vision therapy." Vision therapy consists of a set of treatments over several weeks that combines light and ocular-muscle exercises. What I basically learned was how to look without straining and how to teach my focusing muscles to relax. It is biofeedback training for the eye muscles. Happily for me, it worked. While my nearsightedness was never severe, it lessened by 40 percent. I am now only two lines on the eye chart away from getting my driver's license without glasses. But even more important to me than the improvement in my vision was what I learned about how I see.

How I see with my physical eyes functionally varies with my inner vision. Fluctuations are sometimes small, sometimes dramatic. When I am pushing myself and hurrying from activity to activity, not seeing the bigger picture of life, physically I cannot clearly see as far. When I relax and am less fearful, more present in the moment, my distance vision improves. The big picture is clearer.

Farsightedness involves the opposite process.

Instead of the eyes, straining and pushing out, they retreat and pull in. You can't see what is too close if you are farsighted. What is hard to see clearly is right in front of you and yet too near for clarity. While farsightedness may just mean you are reaching good old middle age, it might mean more. Consider whether you might be having trouble getting a focus on relationships with those closest to you. Are you retreating from seeing something? Is there something happening inside yourself you would rather not see? The big picture on the horizon of your life may be clear but the present very fuzzy.

Suzanna couldn't see clearly even with corrective lenses. Things were always a bit blurry around the edges. Interestingly, her glasses had rose-colored lenses, but that didn't make life look any brighter to her. In fact, Suzanna couldn't see any future at all for herself. She couldn't envision herself in the years to come, couldn't see herself marrying, having kids, growing old—nothing. After she did hard personal work—psychotherapy, spiritual work, and body therapy—an invitation came to Suzanna that she decided to risk accepting.

A friend told Suzanna about the eye surgery he was going to have. The surgery, Photorefractive-Keratectomy (PRK), is laser eye surgery for vision problems that cannot be corrected with glasses or contact lenses. Just recently approved in this country, the surgery has been done for many years in Europe. This man was going to London with his American ophthalmologist to have the surgery. Did Suzanna want to look into going with him and having it done? Such an invitation is hardly one most people would jump at. Suzanna is a careful person and spent a good bit of time with the American doctor, asking many questions and reading literature. She decided to do it.

What followed were several days of roller-coaster feelings. She was excited about the possibility of seeing clearly for the first time in her life, at least out of one eye, because only one eye can be operated on at a time. Terror replaced excitement during the surgery. What if she was blinded by this? There was considerable pain following the surgery and relief as the medications, balms, and ministrations of the ophthalmologist worked. Within days, she could see the outlines of objects and people in clear focus for the first time in her memory. But she could see clearly only out of her right eye. The left eye still saw the world the way it always had.

"I feel like I saw the world from two levels, actually and emotionally. With one eye, the world looked the way it always had. With the other, the whole world seemed different. I can't describe it, but I knew some-how I had changed, not just my eyes." Suzanna became acutely aware of how vulnerable she felt without glasses on her face. She felt exposed, naked even, that people could now see how she felt.

A contact lens for the non-treated eye adjusted Suzanna's vision until she had surgery on the other eye three months later. That helped her feel less unbalanced visually. Regaining her balance emotionally took more time. She realized how hard it is to get motivated when you can't see clearly, when it's all a blur, as it had been all her life. The depression she had suffered since adolescence took on a new meaning. She understood the struggle she had faced every day in just seeing where she was going and what was happening.

Seeing clearly now meant she was much more present to what and who was around her. Life looked real, and she knew with more certainty that she was a part of it. Getting used to being exposed and vulnerable isn't easy. It's too soon to know for sure what Suzanna will see with clarity in the future. There's no doubt, though, that her whole world looks different.

Genetics, diet, fatigue, stress, and disease all play a role in eye problems. These factors are not to be denied nor minimized when it comes to diagnosing eye problems. But there is much more than the physical involved in seeing, even in seeing light. Listen to what Jacques Lusseyran, who was blinded at age seven, sees: "At that time I still wanted to use my eyes. I followed their usual path. I looked in the direction where I was in the habit of seeing before the accident. ... Finally, I realized that I was looking in the wrong way. I was looking too far off, and too much on the surface of things. ... I began to look more closely, not at things but at a world closer to myself, looking from an inner place to one further within, instead of clinging to the movement of sight toward the world outside. Immediately, the substance of the universe drew together, redefined and peopled itself anew. I was aware of a radiance emanating from a place I knew nothing about, a place which might as well have been outside me as within. ... I felt indescribable relief, and happiness so great it almost made me laugh. ... Sighted people always talk about the night of blindness, and that seems to them quite natural. But there is no such night, for at every waking hour and even in my dreams I lived in a stream of light. Without my eyes, light was much more stable than it had been with them. As I remember it, there was no longer the same difference between things lighted brightly, less brightly, or not at all. I saw the whole world in light, existing through it and because of it."

I invite you to consider more than the physical mechanisms of vision when you think of how you see. The exercises below are designed to help you in that process of discovery.

The following exercise is a Hatha Yoga technique that helps stretch and loosen the muscles around the eyes. Be gentle with yourself as you do this. Don't strain or push. Remember that disrupting a fixed pattern of viewing life can be unsettling emotionally. Simply take note of what you experience or remember. Stop if it becomes too uncomfortable for you, and go back to this exercise at another time. The exercise is vigorous enough that it should not be repeated more than twice a day.

Exercise: Eye Stretching

The goal of this *Eye Stretching* exercise is to contract and stretch the muscles of the eyes by moving them in various directions and holding them as far as they will go in each direction for several seconds. In each position, move the eyes as far as they will go without pain. The positions, with one exception, are paired. That means after looking in one direction, look in the opposite direction. Breathing deeply, begin by holding each position three to five seconds. You can gradually increase the time until each position can be held for half a minute or longer.

Positions

1. Squeeze eyes shut tightly.
2. Now open them as widely as possible.
3. Move your eyes all the way to the left.
4. Move your eyes all the way to the right.
5. Look up toward your eyebrows.
6. Look down at your cheekbones.
7. Cross your eyes so you are looking at the sides of your nose.
8. With your eyes *closed,* rotate them in a clockwise direction several times, making as large circles as possible.
9. Again with your eyes *closed,* rotate the eyes an equal number of times in the opposite direction.
   Notice any emotional reactions or memories that

come into your awareness. Simply observe them, not judging or resisting. If you don't get any pictures or feelings, that's fine, too. Nothing is "supposed to" happen, even though your eye muscles are being gradually stretched and loosened.

The next exercise brings about more immediate results. It's helpful if you're dissociating or having an overwhelming memory/feeling. At times when you might be feeling disconnected from your body and want to get back in it quickly, this exercise will help you do that. Almost immediately you will come back to yourself. It's safe, simple, and quick. You don't have to be in distress to benefit from this exercise. How you see will be expanded no matter what point you start from.

Exercise: Being Present in Your Looking

Pick an object to focus on. It can be a pen, a box of tissues, an apple, your cat, anything actually. Hold it and really look at it. Look at it as if you were going to have to describe it to a blind person. See the lines and the shapes and the shadows and the colors in every detail. Let your eyes focus on this object in a clear, seeing way but without straining. If you find your eyes glazing over, blink a few times and go back to careful looking. Look for one to three minutes. Your eyes will feel different from the way they did when you started this exercise. Your perception probably will be much clearer, and you might notice that you can actually see those things around you a little bit better.

I described what I learned about myself from my nearsightedness vision therapy. This next exercise will give you an opportunity to see (no pun intended) what you discover for yourself when you look in nearsighted and farsighted ways.

Exercise: Nearsighted/Farsighted

If you have on glasses, take them off. Notice what you feel without your glasses. It might be fear or perhaps confusion. Now push your eyes way out, like you are straining to see. Really push. Look real hard. Notice what the pushing does to your body. Try to look around a little with your eyes pushed out. After thirty seconds, stop. Relax your eyes. Shake your head a little. Take a deep breath.

Now do the opposite. Make your eyes retreat so that you are almost pulling them back in your head, narrowing your focus, as if your eyes do not want to see. Again notice what happens to your breathing and what you feel when you do this. Compare the sensation and experience to what you felt with your eyes pushed out versus pulled in. After thirty seconds relax your eyes. Close them gently. Take another deep breath.

Rub your hands together till they get hot, and put them over your eyes. Roll your eyes ten times to the right and ten times to the left. Roll the eyes under the palms, not the palms on the eyes. This last step helps your eyes to recover from the strain of the exercise.

What we see and how we see are powerful forces affecting our bodies. The more we can wake up to our seeing, the more opportunity we have to be aware of that force. If I am angry at what I see, my body is responding to my anger. The muscles tense. Breath gets shallow. My jaw tightens. I'm ready to attack, all because of how I see and how I judge what I see.

My first therapist tells this story on herself. She's from Michigan and never saw a roach until she moved to Texas, not a real roach, those huge, shiny, black, two-inch monsters that can fly. When she first saw one, she thought it was a beetle and wasn't too bothered. Then someone broke the hard truth to her. Those black things running across her kitchen floor at night were roaches. She was furious.

This woman is a meticulous housekeeper, especially when it comes to cleanliness. No roach was going

to insult her standards of housekeeping by marching across her floor. The next roach she saw became Public Enemy Number One. She went after it with a broom (which actually isn't a very efficient way to kill a roach but was an appropriate expression of her sentiment).

She flailed at it mercilessly, getting madder and madder with each blow. Suddenly she stopped. The roach was pretty well done in by this time anyway. She had a revelation: "I don't have to be angry to kill the roach!" She smiled, began to giggle, then erupted in such laughter she had to sit down on the floor. Holding her sides, tears running down her face, viewing the body of her recently demised six-legged enemy, she knew she got it. From that morning on, she saw roaches without anger—same roaches, their descendants, anyway, no anger. It's all in how you see.

This last exercise will give you some practice in becoming aware of the connections between what you see and how you react mentally, emotionally, and physically. Do it once at week at least. It doesn't require any extra time. You can do it while you're doing anything else. Eventually you will start seeing very precisely how you see.

Exercise: Taking It All In

Look around the room you are in for about sixty seconds. Just look. Notice everything you can notice in that time. Pretend you're going to have a pop quiz on the room at the end of one minute.

Now close your eyes and think of the room. What can you remember? What did you see that you hadn't noticed about the room before? What judgments did you have about the room? Were they new judgments or familiar ones? What feelings did you have with what you saw? Mad, scared, bored, irritated, delighted, discouraged? Did your feelings change after you spent one minute truly looking at the environment surrounding you? What did you want to do after you really looked? Run? Change something? Stay longer? Did you do something? Notice how your judgments, feelings, and actions seem to be connected. Just notice. Don't try to change anything. Don't judge yourself. Just seeing how you see changes how you see. The reverse is also true: Changing alters how we see.

When I was in my twenties and going to school on the East Coast, I occasionally spent weekends in New York City. New York City is a great place for people-watching. Just about every version of human being is somewhere on the streets of New York, but I actually saw very few of them. Walking past hundreds of people, I was so filled with fear that I couldn't really look at any of them. I walked with my eyes focused on the sidewalk in front of me. Many people walk through life that way: fearful, averted eyes missing the spectacle of life playing out in front of them. The exercise you just did, *Taking It All In,* can be helpful to you in seeing how your perception of life around you is changing as you change and heal. Do it regularly. You will be amazed at what you discover.

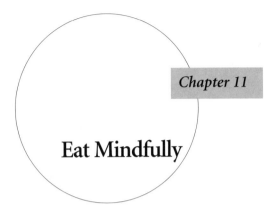

Chapter 11

Eat Mindfully

"Fat coats my nervous system. It numbs the pain."
—*Food Writer*

At any given moment, 48 million people in this country are dieting. The diet industry is a $33 billion a year business. Something is dreadfully wrong with how people in this country eat. Therapists Jane Hirschmann and Carol Munter, experts on compulsive overeating, explain the problem in part this way: "You eat more food than your body requires. You reach for food when you are not physiologically hungry, and if you start out hungry, you continue to eat past the point of physical satiation." People eat food they don't need, and don't actually taste much of the food they do eat. They and we eat mindlessly. Mindful eating is being present and conscious to the experience of consuming food, every moment of it, not just the first and last bites. It is hardly surprising that obesity

211

is such a problem in our nation. Sixty percent of Americans are overweight. We have the greatest fat problem in the history of the world. If you are not present in your body to the experience of eating, how can you possibly know if you are hungry or full? Obesity is a complicated bio-psycho-social problem, but unconscious eating is a contributing factor.

It's a tragedy that so much of the pleasurable experience of eating and tasting food is missed because people have lost the innate ability simply to be present. All babies eat mindfully. As infants, we start out with a remarkable mechanism that enables us to know when we are hungry and/or full. Hungry, we cry until we are fed. Full, we stop eating. Many things happen in people's lives that interfere with this natural response to needing food. In treating compulsive overeaters, one of the first steps is re-establishing the awareness of the body's response to hunger. One way is by learning to differentiate between stomach hunger, and mouth hunger.

Stomach hunger is physiological hunger. It is what we came into the world knowing how to identify. It reflects a physical need to give our bodies fuel. Mouth hunger is psychological hunger. It comes for many reasons: desiring to taste a certain food, wanting to chew or bite, fear of not having enough food later, guilt (about leaving food uneaten or hurting someone's feelings), wanting to soothe ourselves, stuffing emotions back inside, rebellion. The list is long, but the point is that mouth hunger is *not* about the body's need for food.

Eating only in response to mouth hunger is being out of touch with your body. The more you recover your body and learn to eat mindfully, the easier it will be for you to differentiate between stomach and mouth hunger. You may still decide to eat when what you are needing to do is yell or kiss. You'll know the difference, though, and know you are making an informed choice.

Babies and small children participate wholly in eating. They feel their food with their hands or on their faces and are captivated by the sensuous gratification of food. While this is not an endorsement for abandoning all the hard-learned rules of polite gustatory etiquette, it is an urging to consider reclaiming some of that joy children feel from the gift of eating.

Eating can be an icon. An icon is an object or representation of something more. That "something more" can be peace, harmony, union. Every meal or any meal can be an icon if we are willing for it to be so. It doesn't take much. No fancy food is necessary. My morning bowl of granola with maple yogurt and fresh raspberries is an icon of God. When I put down the newspaper and truly taste the sweetness, creaminess, and crunchy texture, I feel gratitude. I wonder why I don't eat every meal that way. I don't, though I am grateful for the times when I do. It makes no difference whether you are munching tortilla chips or savoring a gourmet meal in an elegant restaurant, every eating can be a blessing and a joy.

Eating or drinking mindfully centers and grounds

us. My client Janie has two little kids, ages four and two. One afternoon she was in a hurry to get them fed. She turned on the burner of the gas stove. It wouldn't light. She tried the one beside it. No action. With mounting exasperation she turned on both back burners. Nothing. As fate and planning would have it, there are two stoves in Janie's kitchen. She turned on the backup stove. Nothing! Only gas. No flame. The kids were starting to cry. "Nobody ever plays with me!" wailed the youngest. Clenching her jaw to stop from wailing herself, Janie threw open the three last burners. The smelly hiss of gas and the screams of her kids were all she heard.

Janie is a recovering alcoholic. She still battles internal and external chaos daily. Many times she feels she's "losing it." This was one of those times. Janie turned to her sister Lisa, who is part of Janie's chaos, and said, "I've got to get out of here a minute. I'm going to the grocery store."

She got into the car thinking, "If I could just get a cup of coffee. No, that will take too long." So instead, she drove to a nearby health food store for the groceries she needed. She got what she wanted out of the dairy case and turned to leave. Right in front of her in the store was a coffee bar. "Could you make a decaf cappuccino on ice?" she asked the pony-tailed fellow behind the bar. "I've never done it, but I will," he replied. She sat on the tall wooden stool, her arms on the counter, and waited. He handed her the icy glass with a straw. No glass of wine ever tasted better to her than that cappuccino. Later she told me that as she drank her coffee, "I could feel it going all through me and I knew I'd be all right. Everything was OK. It felt as if I'd been away from the problem a long time." When Janie got home, one burner on one of the stoves lit. They had a good dinner.

Once a day or even once a week, eat a meal without combining it with any other activity. This means not reading, opening the mail, talking on the phone, or even visiting during that time. Just eat. Eat with awareness, tasting each bite of what is going into your body. Eating mindfully will bring you back home to your body, if only for those few minutes. By letting yourself actually savor the food and experiencing whatever you are eating, you will feel satisfied. Be present for the whole thing. Americans have become so driven in their need to be *doing* that the act of daily nourishing the body with food is sometimes treated as a bothersome task to be completed as quickly as possible. Both the body and the psyche pay dearly for the time stolen from this life-sustaining task of eating.

People have become absentee eaters. They are there for the taking but not really involved. If you are an absentee eater, you have had the experience of eating and then realizing that you did not even notice that you had eaten. One of my clients, in reporting on her harried life, said she had been eating her sandwich while she was talking on the phone. "I hung up and looked down and saw my empty plate. I knew I must have eaten my sandwich, but I had absolutely no memory of it. I don't even know how it tasted." Lost satisfaction. That's one meal she'll never eat again, and she missed it completely. Maybe missing out on one of life's moments isn't such a big deal, but add them up and you end up missing out on a pretty big chunk of your life, a potentially very pleasurable chunk.

I went to a nine-day silent meditation retreat where there was no talking, no reading or writing, little sleep, and two modest meals a day. Basically, we meditated from about 5:00 in the morning to 10:00 at night, either in sitting or walking meditation. Meals were understandably a big treat. We really wanted to notice what we were eating, because it would be long hours before food appeared again. Each meal became almost sacramental, consumed in silence and with great appreciation. Lifting the fork, putting the food in the mouth, tasting, and chewing were all conscious parts of the ritual. Making at least one meal a day sacramental brings us in touch with the ancient ritual of being fed. It might even move you a little closer to enlightenment. There is a Zen story in which a disciple asked his master,

"Master, how do you put enlightenment into action? How do you practice it in everyday life?"

"By eating and by sleeping," replied the master.

"But Master, everybody sleeps and everybody eats."

"But not everybody eats when they eat, and not

everybody sleeps when they sleep."

From this comes the famous Zen saying, "When I eat, I eat; when I sleep, I sleep!" This means to be completely present in all your actions.

This next exercise, from Geneen Roth, author of *Breaking Free from Compulsive Eating,* offers helpful suggestions on coming back into your body even before you begin to eat, and knowing when to stop. It will help you be more present to the physical sensations of hunger.

Exercise: Body Check/Hunger Check

Begin by paying careful attention to the bodily sensations that you recognize as hunger. When you feel yourself starting to get hungry, sit down for a few minutes (if you can't sit down, stand still). Where in your body do you experience hunger? In your throat? Your chest? Your stomach? Your legs? How is this sensation different from the sensation, let's say, of excitement? Or loneliness? What happens to you when you feel yourself getting hungry? Do you feel that you need to eat immediately?

When you've decided you are hungry, rate your hunger on a scale of 1 to 10. Rating your hunger numerically provides objective criteria with which to compare past hunger and present hunger. It gives you direct access to an experience that is very subjective and laden with emotional overtones. The low end of the scale can be used to signify "ravenous, very hungry," to "medium," to "just-a-little-hungry." Five is comfortable; at 6, you're starting to get full. When you hit 10, you're up to your neck in food. When you start getting hungry, ask yourself where on the scale the hunger is located. At 5 or above, you probably want to be hungry more than you actually are. Notice the number at which you feel most comfortable eating and the point at which your hunger is uncomfortable.

Listen for the small, quiet voice that says "I've had enough." The difference between hunger and enoughness can be, and often is, a bite, or maybe two. If you are quiet enough and not directing your attention elsewhere, you can hear the body's transition to satisfaction. When you have had enough, it's as if a door latches, something clicks. Your body is saying, "I've had enough. You can keep eating if you want, but I'm ready to stop." That voice is quiet and easy to miss, especially when you aren't used to hearing it or when the food tastes so good you don't want to hear it.

I like Ms. Roth's exercise because it instructs us in mindful eating even before we lift a fork, as well as teaching mindfulness about the physiological sensations of hunger. Once you have food in front of you, the first step in mindful eating is simply seeing the food and noting that you are seeing it.

Notice your goal to take the food; the movement of

your arm, hand, or utensil touching the food lifting your arm; and go on from there, staying with each part of the experience of eating. Try not to miss any of it. Pay attention to your thoughts about the food (anticipation, greed, dissatisfaction, surprise, boredom); the movements of your body as you eat (seeing, lifting the arm, chewing, swallowing); and the sensations of the food (smell, temperature, varieties and changes in taste, fullness in the stomach). If you finish each mouthful before reaching for another, you become more sensitive to your body's needs. One Buddhist teacher observes, "It's very hard to overeat when you eat mindfully."

Try this next exercise sometime when you aren't very hungry. You'll be more patient then. Keep practicing it, at least once a week, and you'll find that within a few weeks all your eating is more mindful. Since it's easy to fall back into old habits, keep doing this exercise occasionally even when you routinely eat mindfully.

Exercise: Notice the Food

Get some food you enjoy—a piece of fruit, a cookie, popcorn, some ice cream. Put it in front of you. Look at the food. Notice the color and the shape. At the same time, be aware of your thoughts and feelings as the food sits before you. What are you feeling? Longing, guilt, eagerness, impatience? Touch the food. Feel the temperature and texture with your finger. Yes, even ice cream. Smell the food. What thoughts come up? Notice changes in your body. Are you salivating more? Is your body tensing? What expression is on your face?

Put the food to your mouth. Feel the movement of your arm and fingers as you do so. Feel your mouth opening. Focus on the sensations of taste. What are you thinking and feeling now? Is there eagerness or even greed to get the next spoonful or bite of sensation to your mouth? Are your thoughts rushing ahead to the next experience and missing this biteful? Are you feeling upset (angry, impatient, bored) with not being able to just eat it and be done with this, not being able to have what you want right away? Are you shaming yourself for wanting or eating the food? Is there disappointment that the food didn't meet your expectation? Were you surprised that it was so good or different?

Continue to chew and swallow, noticing changes in sensation and thought. Note the feel of your jaws as you chew. Now repeat the process with another bite, trying to stay very present to your minute movements, thoughts, sensations of the mouth and body. Be aware of changes in all these areas, how the surprise of taste changes to expectation, how longing changes to satiation (or regret that the food is almost gone). Notice all the many thoughts and feelings that are bound up with this simple process of eating. Don't analyze or try to figure out what this means. Simply notice what you notice as you eat mindfully, with awareness.

A surefire way to become more mindful in your eating is not to eat for a day or part of a day. Fasting may not seem to have much to do with eating mindfully, but it does. When you consciously make the decision to skip a couple of meals, you can become very aware of how your body and your mind respond to food and the lack of it. Fasting has been prescribed by most all of the world's major religions for thousands of years. It must be a good idea to have held on so tenaciously. Sacrifice, giving up something that we want as an offering to God, is one of the spiritual reasons for fasting. Learning nonattachment and breaking free of our grasping habits is another. But separate from any religious precept, fasting is terrific for learning what happens to you when you shake up your eating routine.

Fasting is not dieting. You don't fast in order to make something happen. With a brief fast of a day or so, nothing much will happen externally. You won't look thinner or weigh much less. Your eyes might be a little brighter, but that's beside the point. Fasting is not about willpower, although it takes commitment to the decision not to eat in order to fast. It is not about becoming more virtuous, noble, or spiritual, even though that might happen, too. Fasting is very internal and private. Jesus taught, "When you fast, do not look somber as the hypocrites do, for they disfigure their faces to show men they are fasting. ... But when you fast, put oil on your head and wash your face, so that it will not be obvious to men that you are fasting." Discovery is the goal of fasting.

In my religion, two days of fasting a year are recommended: Ash Wednesday and Good Friday. I look forward to those days. They feel like days of freedom and insight to me. I like having a break from thinking about what I'll eat for breakfast, lunch, and dinner, and I am always curious about how my body and I will get along without the usual regime. I also fast if I'm at an all-day meditation. You don't need much food when you meditate. What feeds you seems to come from something else. The other time I fast is when I'm starting something big, like an intensive writing stretch. Letting go of solid food for a day seems to free me up for whatever else I have to do.

The sweet part is that when your day of fasting is over, you have the divine reward of eating again. Those first few bites of food will be mindful ones, and perhaps all your eating for a while thereafter will be more so. I always end a fast with a greater reverence and appreciation for food. Even the simplest food tastes sublime after an abstinence.

Fasting doesn't have to be often or long or anguishing. It definitely shouldn't cause suffering. A little discomfort is OK, but no misery. If you have any questions about whether or not a brief fast would be detrimental to your health, check with your physician. The next exercise explains one way to fast.

Exercise: Not Eating to Eat Mindfully

Decide ahead of time when you are going to fast. I usually know days or weeks ahead that a certain day will be a fast-day for me. Knowing ahead helps us prepare for the period of deprivation. You might decide to eat a little more on the day or night before you begin your fast, or you might not. It doesn't matter. How long you fast is up to you. Again, decide ahead. If it's your first time to fast, going without breakfast and lunch may be enough. If you want to go a full day and night, that's OK, too. The main thing is that you know this is going to happen.

The morning you start your fast, have a glass of fruit juice. Orange juice is probably not the best choice, because it has too much acid and sugar to work well on an empty stomach. If you have a juicer at home, make whatever kind of juice you like. If you are buying juices for the day, buy the kind that health food stores have, such as unfiltered apple juice, the cloudy kind. Get your juices and some lemons the day before you start.

The rest is simple. Drink juices or water with fresh lemon in it anytime you want—all day, during the evening, whenever. If you start to feel a little weak, drink some juice. When you get hungry, first have some "lemon water," hot or cold, then drink some more juice. Don't limit yourself. I always have on hand more juice than I can drink, and I usually have a couple of choices so that I don't get bored with the same juice all day.

Make up your mind that you will stick with it. You won't die from the discomfort, although you might think more about people who are actually dying from hunger. Just stick it out with awareness. Pay attention to the sensations of your body and to all the thoughts and feelings that come up about food or anything else. Don't try to ignore any of it. There's no point in fasting if you do it obliviously. Be awake to the contractions, grumbling (of your mind and stomach), longing, fear. Note it all. Take a soaking bath or shower at the end of your fasting day if you can. It helps.

When your fast time is up, give thanks for your discoveries and the food with which you "break fast." Eat lightly. Your stomach has shrunk a little. Your mind and mouth have more longing for food at this point than your body does. Enjoy. You did it, and you recovered a bit more of your body.

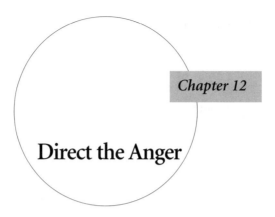

Chapter 12

Direct the Anger

"Just as physical pain tells us to take our hand
off the hot stove, the pain of our anger preserves
the very integrity of our self."
—*Harriet Goldhor Lerner*

Anger is not bad. Writer Julia Cameron says, "Anger is the firestorm that signals the death of our old life. Anger is the fuel that propels us into our new one. Anger is a tool, not a master." The trick is to learn to manage anger so that it is indeed a tool and doesn't become a firestorm that destroys us or others. How we use anger is a choice, and we all have a responsibility to learn to manage it appropriately. Thomas Merton, the Christian mystic monk, understood anger. He said: "A temperamentally angry man may be more inclined to anger than another. But as long as he remains sane, he is still free not to be angry. His inclination to anger is simply a force in his character which can be turned to good or evil, according to his desires. If he desires what is evil, his temper will become a weapon of evil against other men and even against his own soul. If he desires what is good, his temper can become the controlled instrument for fighting the evil that is in himself and helping other men to overcome the obstacles which they meet in the world. He remains free to desire either good or evil."

Problems with anger can come from holding in too much or too little. Raging people have trouble experiencing feelings other than anger. People who fear anger, their own and others', have difficulty accepting anger as a natural, and at times necessary, human response. Both are out of touch with bodily responses to the blocked emotions. People who rage often are unaware of feelings of fear, sadness, or helplessness in their bodies. At the other end of the spectrum are people who deny their anger and attribute their headaches and tight shoulders to tension.

There's no right way to be angry. What is helpful to one may be harmful to another. Research done at the University of British Columbia in Vancouver found that venting anger while under stress has opposite effects on the blood pressure of men and women. Expressing hostility seems to lower men's blood pressure, but women seem to lower their blood pressure by holding it in. In another study, men who already had high blood pressure raised it even more if they held in their anger under stress. It didn't work that way for women. Some studies have found that women who hold in their anger recover normal blood pressure much more rapidly than women who vent hostility after stress.

How old you are may influence how you handle your anger. Sandra Thomas, who has done the first large investigation of women's anger, found that the younger the woman, the more likely she was to feel and express anger. Women over fifty-five reported the least anger and were most likely to suppress the feeling. Those in their forties experienced the most physical symptoms from anger. Crying was the number one physical reaction to fury. The women who appeared most successful at coping with anger were those who talked about their feelings.

So be respectful of your own history and learn from your body what works for you. But when anger comes up, it is essential to have coping strategies that will not hurt you or someone else. Sometimes just acknowledging that you are angry is all that is necessary, especially if you came from a family where anger was not allowed or never expressed. "Rageaholics" fail to contain their angry emotional response, and literally explode. Those at the opposite extreme fail to release sufficiently for a natural balancing. Obviously, the work each of these types needs to do to recover the body is not the same.

Awareness is the approach found most successful in helping rageful people not to use their anger as a weapon. If you are a rager, you can learn to recognize inflaming self-talk and biological changes that indicate mounting anger, such as more rapid breathing, a clenched jaw, and heat from flushing. Once you recognize the anger symptoms, you can learn to respond differently to the cues. For rageaholics, trying to work out anger by expressing it is like trying to put out a fire by pouring gasoline on the flames. The fire rapidly gets out of control. Instead the rager must learn to transcend or dissolve any angry feelings before they take over. A Zen saying applies here: "The occurrence of an evil thought is a malady; not to continue it is the remedy."

Something of the opposite is required of people who fear anger. For them the "hydraulic" theory of anger might apply. This theory assumes that anger mounts until it is released, and if not released, the built-up tension can cause various negative consequences for the body, including heart disease, high blood pressure, rashes, strokes, cancer, and arthritis. It is not that simple, of course. Our moods, beliefs, and attitudes do have powerful effects on our bodies, but the expression or holding in of anger is not the sole determinant of physical or mental well-being.

The first exercises in this chapter are for those of you who are "hot tempered" and who readily react with anger. Newton Hightower, a social worker who successfully has taught both violent offenders and ordinary people how to control and transcend their rage, developed the *Ten Anger Management* techniques given here.

They work, but only if you do them. So do them. Your relationships with others, and maybe even with your own life, are at stake.

The second set of exercises is for those of you who have trouble feeling and expressing your own anger and being around others who are angry. In some households, it's as if there is a sign over the kitchen door declaring, *"No Anger Allowed!"* My house was sort of like that. It took me quite a while to learn to be honest about my anger and to express it with integrity. The exercises in the last part of this chapter will help you to feel safer with anger.

Ten Anger Management Exercises

The first requirement in managing your anger is admitting that it is an addiction and is self-stimulating. This means acknowledging that you are an "adrenaline junkie" and that the adrenaline rush has become your way of coping with life's difficulties. The next requirement is to commit to "abstinence," which means discontinuing all expressions of anger. If you are willing to meet those two prerequisites, which, admittedly, take courage, you are on your way and ready to begin the exercises. Here are the steps:

1. Practice silence.
Whenever anyone does or says anything you don't like, remain silent.

2. Get out.

Leave a situation before you get out of control. This leaving is called "time out," not cowardice.

3. Allow interruptions.

If someone stops you while you are still talking or making your point, go back to #1, assuming silence.

4. Break eye contact.

Animal researchers have found that a low-ranking member avoids confrontation with the dominant one by turning away from the dominant animal's stare and adopting a crouching position. Be willing to relinquish the dominant position in a conflict. Stop your challenging look and break eye contact. Try putting your elbows on your knees when you look away. You'll see that immediately the violent tension, yours and the other person's, will lessen.

5. Renounce violence or threats of violence, even "if" threats.

This means you do not allow yourself to say anything that implies a threat, like "If you say that again, you're asking for it!"

6. Don't shout.

Ask a partner, spouse, or friend to let you know when he or she thinks you are shouting.

7. Don't use profanity.

Cursing is very stimulating and can escalate your anger further. All profane words and foul or abusive language must be edited out of both your speaking and your thinking.

8. Avoid name-calling.

This includes any kind of direct labeling, not just profanity.

9. Don't tell war stories.

"War stories" are tales of previous anger episodes, including those of how you were wronged. They are self-stimulating and have to be stopped.

10. Don't point.

A pointed finger means the blame and responsibility are being pushed off on someone else. Put your hand down and go back to Exercises 1-9 in this section.

This next anger "reorienting" exercise is from Jean Deschener's *The Hitting Habit*. If you rage, practice this exercise once a week and use it anytime you feel yourself losing control of your anger. If you do it regularly, it will be more readily available as part of your mental repertoire for "emergencies."

Exercise: Turn Off the Road to Anger

Allow your eyes to close. Take a deep breath. Hold it for a second and then slowly exhale. After you exhale, let your breathing return to normal. Now take another long, deep breath, feeling first your abdomen, then your chest. Hold the breath for a second or two, then exhale. Let your breathing return to normal when the breath is out. Take one more long, slow, deep breath, feeling again first your abdomen, then your chest. Hold it for a second or two. Now exhale. Allow your breathing to return to normal. Let your body continue to relax. Focus on your jaw muscle. Let it relax. Let the tension go out of your jaw. Let the tension go out of your neck, out of your shoulders. Become more and more relaxed. Continue to let your body relax. Let go and notice how much relaxation you can achieve in just a minute or two, by yourself, with just these simple instructions. Now let yourself become more and more relaxed.

Now imagine that you are standing in the express checkout lane in a busy grocery store on a Saturday afternoon. The sign says clearly, "Limit 10 items, CASH ONLY." You are in a hurry. You're late for an important appointment. You've stopped to pick up a quick snack because you haven't had lunch. You have only two items. The person ahead of you in line not only has more than ten items but begins to get a checkbook out of her purse. Now notice what you are beginning to tell yourself. Instead of continuing to get angry, turn off the road to anger by telling yourself, "This, too, shall pass. Calm down. This, too, shall pass. Calm down. This, too, shall pass."

Now imagine that you are in a movie theater and the feature has just begun. A man and his date start down your row. He's carrying a bag of popcorn and talking to his girlfriend. He steps on your toes and spills the popcorn in your lap and begins laughing. He doesn't apologize. Notice what you tell yourself that is beginning to create irritation, annoyance, or anger. Instead of continuing to make yourself angry, choose to turn off the road to anger by telling yourself, "Calm down. This, too, shall pass. Calm down. This, too, shall pass. Calm down. This, too, shall pass."

Now imagine you're coming out of your house in the morning ready to go to work. You see that your front windshield has been shattered. As you get closer to your car, you see that a brick has been thrown through your front windshield. Notice what kind of self-talk begins. Notice what you tell yourself that creates feelings of anger, hatred, or revenge. Instead of increasing your anger, choose to turn off the road to anger by saying to yourself, "Calm down. This, too, shall pass. Calm down. This, too, shall pass. Calm down. This, too, shall pass." Now if you've been doing this exercise with your eyes closed, allow your eyes to open. Notice the difference in how you feel and notice the change you have made in your breathing, your heart rate, and your emotions in just a few moments. You really can turn off the road to anger.

John Coon, my yoga teacher, shared this "quick cooling" exercise with me. He learned it from his teacher, who said, "Many problems have been solved over a drink—of water."

Exercise: Cooling the Fire with Water

When you are starting to get angry or even already are steaming, take a full glass of water, at least eight ounces—not hot water, not ice cold—room temperature or cool is best. Now drink it "bottoms up," no stopping. Sipping will not do the trick! You will immediately feel calmer.

What happens physiologically with this simple little technique is that the rapid swallowing causes the blood pressure to drop, countering the rise in pressure that comes with anger. The abdomen and throat must relax in order to swallow the water, so the tight muscles in your neck and gut release. Finally, the core of the body is subtly cooled, and you end up more cool-headed, with all the benefits that implies. Isn't it amazing what a simple glass of water can do? Try putting out your fire with it!

Now come the exercises for those of you who are anger phobic or simply don't know what to do with your anger when and if you do feel it. Releasing anger can be as difficult and frightening for some people as holding it back is for rageaholics. In violent households, any expression of anger can signal the beginning of an emotional eruption that can end in physical assault or injury. The formula in raging families is simple: Someone gets mad equals someone/something gets destroyed. In contrast, families that express little or no honest anger give the covert message that anger is to be avoided at all costs. Either way, anger comes to be thought of as some monstrous demon, which, if unleashed, will destroy the entire family or at least some of the people in it. Violent, raging families are scary, but fear-phobic families are frightening in a different way. They tend to be infected with bitterness, rigidity, cynicism, and somatic complaints. It's hard to feel alive in your body when it's carrying so much undischarged feeling.

Children who have been abused rightly fear that any expression of anger will heap further abuse upon them. They carry that fear into adulthood. When Sarah began to do anger-expressive exercises, she was asked to hit a mattress with a tennis racket. This particular exercise is used quite routinely by psychotherapists familiar with bioenergetic exercises. Sarah did the exercise, but the whole time she was hitting, she felt someone was standing behind her, waiting to "get her." It took time for her to feel anger not shadowed by fear. So be patient and kind with yourself if you find these exercises for expressing anger difficult. There is some very good reason you have trouble with anger. Respect your history and the way you learned to survive.

Exercise: Get Off My Back!

Stand up. Bend your elbow. Have your knees

slightly flexed. Now push your elbows back forcefully while saying firmly, or even shouting, "Get off my back. Off! Off! Get off my back. Off. Off." Keep doing this for one to five minutes. Then relax. Sit or lie down. Reflect on what you felt during the exercise and afterwards. The release of pent-up anger may be refreshing or frightening. You may start out serious but end up laughing, or vice-versa. Watch your feelings and body change. Anger you were not aware of may erupt. Just notice it.

End this exercise and the next one with the Golden Light meditation. Doing so will help ease some of the agitation you may feel after releasing "forbidden" feelings. I'll repeat it here in case you have forgotten.

Sit or lie quietly for a minute or two. Invite the healing Golden Light into that part in you that is now and always will be pure. Take a few minutes to find it. Breathe normally, and imagine this warm Golden Light flowing into your pure center with each breath. Just feel or see the Light come, filling your body with soothing energy. As the Light touches and penetrates you, allow it to cleanse and purify all your wounds, pain, suffering, held-in hurts, and shame. Let yourself be dissolved into the Light, even if only for a moment. Rest in this renewing and restoring Light. As the Presence fades, express your "thank you" for the release and slowly rise to go about your business, knowing you are now a little different, a little freer, and a little more recovered in body.

The *No! No! No!* exercise that follows will give you the experience of safely releasing held-in anger. If you locked in your anger years ago, the feeling of letting it be expressed with your whole body can be exhilarating, confusing, or scary. Give it your best shot and see what comes. You can always stop yourself, just as you have much of your life.

Exercise: No! No! No!

The basic movements of this exercise are those of a two-year-old lying on the floor and throwing a temper tantrum. Lie on your back on the bed or on top of pillows on the floor. To avoid bruising or injuring yourself, do not do this exercise on a hard surface.

Bend your knees so that your feet are flat on the floor or bed. Clench your fist. Now let it all out! Stamp your feet, hit the floor/bed with your fists, and move your head from side to side. As you do this, say or yell, as loudly as you can, "No! No! No!" Keep doing it as long as you can, ideally for ten to twenty minutes. Move your arms, legs, and head as rapidly and vigorously as feels safe to you. Try to keep your neck from arching backward or forward. If you need to rest, stop briefly and then continue. Try to establish a rhythm and then speed up as you feel emotions coming up. Don't flail, but rather keep the movements contained to the point where you do not feel swept away. Keep moving as long as you can for up to twenty minutes.

You don't have to do this exercise for twenty minutes, but if you find you're stopping quickly, push on a little longer. Stopping quickly may mean you just reached the edge of the anger and are afraid of it. Unrecognized anger can quickly surface once the body's restrictions are freed.

End with the healing Golden Light meditation given at the end of the previous exercise.

CAUTION: As I said before, this exercise is not appropriate for people who have trouble controlling their anger. If you have an anger addiction, this exercise will only give you a "fix." You won't be any more recovered in body, mind, or spirit for doing it.

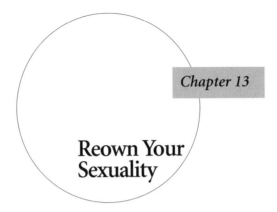

Chapter 13

Reown Your Sexuality

"Sex is difficult; yes. But those tasks that have been
    entrusted to us are difficult; almost everything serious
    is difficult; and everything is serious."
                                            —*Rainer Maria Rilke*

S ex is tricky. It can be an expression of the Divine
or a profanity of the soul. When you lose your
body, one of the first things to go may be sex, or it
may be the last vestige of physical aliveness when everything else goes dead. If you were sexually abused as a
child or raped as an adult, your sexual responsiveness is
complicated by those experiences. Even without abuse,
it is a rare person who feels a natural ease with sexuality. Most of us carry at best some ambivalence about it.

Our bodies can betray us sexually. I have had clients
who reported, with great shame, that they felt sexual
arousal and pleasure while they were being mastur-
bated incestuously. At the same moment they were

emotionally recoiling, their bodies were responding positively to the stimulation. Some of them never trusted their sexuality, or their bodies, after that. They simply quit having sexual feelings and learned to live with the loss. For them, feeling sexual wasn't worth the risk of betrayal. Their sexual feelings were simply too dangerous to be trusted.

And yet to ignore sexual arousal and impulses in our bodies is like trying to ignore a jungle cat shut up in the next room. Sexual energy is one of the most powerful forces in the body. It must have needed to be that way for our species's survival. What it takes to suppress or ignore that energy is a great deal of counterforce, which can take the form of physical or mental rigidity. Stiffening up is one way to numb your sexuality. But when you start breathing and moving, as you know by now, that rigidity begins to break up, and you are likely to be confronted with long-forgotten sexual feelings.

Reowning sexuality has nothing to do with having sex with someone else. You don't ever have to have sex with another person to be sexually alive. Intercourse and other sexual behaviors are expressions of sexuality. You can behave sexually and still feel sexually dead, or you can be celibate and sexually alive. Acting sexually and feeling sexual energy are not the same, even though they can and do happen at the same time. This chapter is about reclaiming a natural part of your body's aliveness. It is not a prescription for or a proscription against interpersonal behavior, sexual or celibate. Poet Andrew Harvey, who spent years immersing himself in intensive meditation study, confesses, "I've had all the out-of-body experiences that an accomplished escapee can have. I've seen flashing lights of every kind. But what I'm really just beginning to have is the in-body experience—of the integration of the light with every moment of ordinary life—including the radiance and holiness of sexuality, the sacredness of sexuality." The work in this chapter is about being in a sacredly sexual body.

Like exercise or food or work, sex can be an addiction. It can keep you for a time from feeling pain. Sex becomes a symbol of being loved, desired, wanted—a desperate defense against unlovableness. A quick flipping through the fashion magazines brings home how willing we are to buy whatever implies the promise of sex. Unfortunately, addictive sex in an unrecovered body is like a misting rain shower on parched ground. It helps soften the surface for a few minutes but doesn't change the basic aridity. Sexual energy can be transforming only if it is experienced in a physically and emotionally alive body.

How you transform your sexual energy depends on both your history and your goals. I have a client who considers a day incomplete if she and her partner haven't had sex. Sex for her is a form of reassurance and closeness. She uses it as affirmation. Others use it for creative expression or to move closer to a sense of oneness with God. Whatever the intent or the expression, sexual aliveness begins with honoring and experiencing it through the sense of touch.

This next exercise may feel nurturing or terrifying, depending upon where you are with your sexuality. Do what you feel you can do. Don't force it. If just reading the exercise makes you recoil in fear, leave it alone for now and come back to it when you feel more ready.

Exercise: Honoring Your Sensuality

Set aside half an hour when you won't be disturbed. Fill a bathtub with water exactly the temperature you like. (You can do this exercise in a shower if you don't have a tub.) Pour in some bath salts or oil while the tub is filling. Baking soda, seasalt, baby oil, or even apple cider vinegar will do if you don't have any special salts or oils.

Very slowly and carefully undress yourself, as if you are being undressed by a lover or a gentle parent. (If any of these steps trigger upsetting memories of abuse, *don't do them*.) Again slowly, step into the tub or shower. Feel the water flow over your skin. Breathe in the smell of the water, salts, or oils. Feel your muscles start to relax and your breath slow. Lie there two or three minutes, just feeling your body in the water. As much as possible keep your thoughts on the physical sensations.

Now reach down and touch one foot. Slowly and firmly rub each toe. Rub the bottom of your foot and the top. Rub between your toes. Don't skip any spot. Put your foot down and take the other foot, rubbing it carefully and lovingly in the same manner. Now move to the ankles of each leg. Proceed up one leg, massaging or just touching the calf, knee, and thigh. Do the same with the other leg. Don't rush.

Move now to the top of your head. Gently rub your scalp, beginning at the crown and working down. Caress your ears, inside and out. Now your face, slowly touching each spot. Move to your neck and shoulders. Give them plenty of time and attention, applying extra pressure where they seem to want it. Reach down on your back as far and you can, stroking it as you reach. If your have a long-handled bath brush, use that to rub all over your back.

From your back, move the touching to your arms. Rub each one with long, firm strokes. Give extra attention to the elbow and wrist joints. Massage each hand, one finger at a time. Rub the palm and the top of the hand, too. Next take your attention back up to your chest.

You are moving into the private zones now, so watch your breath. If it becomes shallow or you find yourself speeding up the touch, slow down and breathe more deeply. Notice if any places feel numb to the touch. If so, don't try to change the sensation. Just be aware of it. Lovingly massage your chest and breasts. Rub them exactly the way you would want to be rubbed. This sensuous touch may bring up those inner-critic voices. Just note them and go back to attending to the sensations.

Now begin to rub your belly with slow, clockwise circles. Rub it firmly but with gentleness. Move to your hips. Massage the upper buttocks first, then the lower part. Give each side equal attention.

By now you may be feeling sexually aroused, anxious, impatient, or bored. Regardless, just acknowledge it and keep going at the same speed, not rushing, not resisting.

The last area of your body to caress is your genitals. Touch them slowly, with awareness, with love. The goal is not to make something happen. It's not to have a sexual climax, although that's fine if it happens. (If you have the sexual addiction problem of compulsive masturbation, try to do this exercise without masturbation. Just tolerate the sexual tension until the exercise is complete.) The intent is to allow yourself to feel the sexual sensations of genital touch in an awakened, loved body. Experiment a little with what kind of pressure or touch feels good to you. Stop when you feel ready.

Slowly get out of the shower or tub. Dry yourself gently. Dress yourself with love. Give praise for your sense-filled, sexual body.

You might have encountered all sorts of barriers in doing this exercise—distractions from phone, family, or your own sense of impatience. Allotting time solely to experiencing your sensuality can bring up pragmatic or puritanical voices you didn't even know were there. If any of those things stopped you from completing the exercise, I urge you to go back to it again and again until you can do the entire process and discover some pleasure in doing it. Once you have internal permission to be sensuously touched all over, you can move on to the next step—kissing.

Kissing? Everyone kisses! Well, yes and no. People kiss at and go through the motions, but not everyone savors the sensation of touching with lips, which is a shame. Our lips give us such an opportunity for expressing and receiving love, caring, kindness, passion, and sentiment. As Diane Ackerman reminds us, "We don't just kiss romantically, of course; we also kiss dice before we roll them, kiss our own hurt finger or that of a loved one, kiss a religious symbol or statue, kiss the flag of our homeland or the ground itself, kiss a good-luck charm, kiss a photograph, kiss the king's or bishop's ring, kiss our own fingers to signal farewell to someone." That's not to mention kissing babies, our kids, parents, pets, spouses, partners, teachers, and friends. The kissing exercise below is a way to wake up to sensual/sexual sensations that you are already having but may be muted.

Exercise: Kissing Yourself Awake

Start by making a commitment to kiss someone or something every day. Kiss whatever you like that will let you do it: your dog, a photo, your own reflection in a mirror, a person, a treasured object. Just make sure you deliver at least one kiss a day. Now, don't just hurriedly kiss to get the assignment over. Kiss with intent. Kissing with intent doesn't mean kissing passionately. It means kissing mindfully, with awareness. Your kiss-for-the-day may be just a peck on someone's cheek, but it needs to be a peck that you experience.

Before you kiss, think a moment about the kiss you are about to deliver. Consider how you feel about giving that kiss. Decide what kind of kiss you want it to be. Prepare yourself to feel it. Be aware of your lips as they change shape as you prepare to kiss. Feel the sensation on your lips as they touch whatever or whomever you kiss. Notice your feelings and body sensations while you kiss and afterwards. In short, don't miss a moment of it. Kiss however you want—long, short, sweet, wet, formal, gentle, passionate. If you like the sensation, you can do it again or keep it going. But remember that only one kiss per day is assigned. If you didn't like it, don't kiss that way or that person/object/pet again. Do this for four weeks. That's twenty-eight kisses. By then you will have awakened your kissing capacity and are ready for the next step in reclaiming your sexuality.

After a month of mindful kissing, you still may not be very crazy about the whole thing. No problem. It may be a problem for those who want to kiss you, but you can now make your kissing decisions with "informed consent." For twenty-eight days, you consented to kiss and you were observant while you were kissing. If you decide to drop kissing from your repertoire of behaviors, so be it. You and the world will manage without your kisses. It is much better by far that you not kiss at all than to kiss or be kissed unwillingly.

Should you decide to keep certain kissing options open, great. It's probably wise not to rule out ever kissing anything/anyone again based on your twenty-eight-day research data. People change in what they want and need. You may change and someday want to kiss or be kissed again. If so, go ahead, but kiss with intent. Kissing is too fraught with possible pleasure to be done obliviously.

You have reawakened your body's sensuality with the first exercise in this chapter. You researched your kissing capacity with the second. The next step is reclaiming embraces. Hugs can be both harder and easier than kisses to give. We can give bear hugs; greeting hugs; reassuring hugs; passionate, lover-type hugs; consoling hugs. Some require intimacy. Some don't. We all have preferences about how we do or don't want to be hugged and by whom, the same as with kisses. But there's no doubt that hugs require us to put at least a little more of our bodies into it than is necessary with a kiss. So part of reclaiming your sexuality is knowing your preferences. This next exercise will help you identify your preferences.

Exercise: Hug-A-Day

Just as with the kissing exercise above, you begin by making the decision to give one hug a day. Hug whatever you want, animate or inanimate, that allows hugs. Mix it up, though, so that sometimes you are hugging something/someone alive and sometimes something not so alive, like a stuffed animal. Don't just hug impulsively, at least not for the assignment. Think about your hug and deliver it with intent. Feel your arms as they move to embrace. Be aware of what you are feeling emotionally about the hug you give. How does your body feel as you hug? And afterwards? If you enjoyed the hug and want more, do it again or keep it going. If you didn't like it, think a moment about what you didn't like about it. Listen to any voices in your head about the hug, how you're doing it, how it ought to be, anything else.

Give one intentional hug a day for four weeks. The purpose of these twenty-eight hugs is not to make you or anyone else feel any better. It's to reawaken your senses to the experience of physical embrace and to remember that you have choice about how you respond to them. Choose what works for you and leave the rest alone, for now anyway.

Sex is not the same thing to everyone. Sex may be like fingerprints—everyone has a unique pattern.

Reclaiming your sexuality begins with knowing what your own pattern is, what pleases you and what feels right for you. If you avoid the whole thing as much as possible, you cheat yourself of knowing that sexual or sensual behavior, like kissing or hugging, might be exactly on the mark for you, emotionally and physically. Likewise, if you plunge into sex impulsively and addictively, you have no way of discriminating what it is about sex that your body needs or wants. Sexual behavior can become contaminated with other motivations, like anger, low self-esteem or fear of abandonment. Reclaiming your sexuality means taking the time to investigate what happens to your body and your emotions when you consciously engage in sensuous activities. Take your time to discover what you may not know about your own sexual responsiveness. Do the three exercises given above repeatedly until you feel truly informed about your sexual pattern. Then move on to whatever you choose to do or not do sexually. Regardless of what you accept or reject, you will be doing it with a different consciousness. You'll be responding from a true knowing of what your body wants, needs, and feels.

Sexual satisfaction is not a matter of how much sex you are getting. I once had a client who would have sex with his girlfriend in the morning and with his wife at night. He was one of the most miserable men I have ever treated. No matter how much sex he was getting, he had no emotional satisfaction. I'm not sure he even had that much physical satisfaction either. Sex for him was a desperate attempt at control, to keep the women from leaving him. He was terrified of being alone. As long as he could have sex with a woman, that demon of loneliness howled and shook but stayed in the dark forest. Using sex that way is dangerous, physically as well as emotionally.

Married men who are having affairs may even be at higher risk of having fatal coronary attacks. Cardiologists Doctors Martin S. Gizzi and Bernard Gitler, of New Rochelle Hospital and Medical Center, only half in jest said that "the contemplation of bigamy" should be listed by the American Heart Association as a risk factor for death from coronary artery disease. They report several cases in which they believe the patient's involvement with more than one woman contributed to coronary distress. In one case, in which a man with two fiancées had a massive heart attack, they suggest that "the man's chaotic sexual life may have been a primary factor in his brush with death from heart disease." Having sex under those conditions of stress has little to do with sexual pleasure in a recovered body. It's kind of a pitiful imitation of what's possible. Don't settle for that kind of sex. You deserve better.

The exercises in this chapter will get you on the road to knowing what's best for your body sexually. Should you find they lead you to an understanding that you have more work to do and need guidance, there are fine therapists who specialize in sex therapy, and helpful books have been written on the subject. Avail yourself of both. Begin, however, with an investigation of your own sexual body by doing these exercises and the others in the book. Any work you do with a therapist will benefit from your having done this basic sexual homework on your own. Try your best not to be afraid, ashamed, or grandiose about your sexual body. Like your ability to receive pleasure from your eyes, ears, and mouth, your sexuality is there as a potential gift, no matter how it has been used or misused in the past.

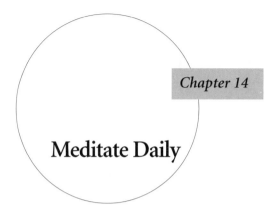

Chapter 14

Meditate Daily

"There are seconds—they come five or six at
a time—when you suddenly feel the presence of
eternal harmony in all its fullness."

—*Dostoevski*

Meditate daily. That recommendation may
seem absurd to those of you who are scarf-
ing down your food and rushing breath-
lessly through each day. But don't dismiss the idea as an
impossibility. There is no more thorough and better
way to reconnect with your body on a daily basis than
to meditate. The benefits for both the body and mind
are well documented. Frequent meditators report significantly fewer stressors and illness symptoms; lower
levels of anxiety, hostility, depression, and dysphoria;
and higher levels of feeling positive than do infrequent
meditators. While the actual number of stressors is
not lower, the frequent meditators perceive themselves

as having fewer stressors and being upset less by those they do have. They are more at peace in the face of adversity. Meditators report having a greater sense of self-worth, not being as easily influenced by others, arriving at decisions more quickly and easily, and being more accepting of themselves and others. The capacity for love is increased, along with greater vitality and efficiency. So at least entertain the possibility of finding a place for meditation in your life.

Meditation is the core of the Stress Reduction Clinic at the University of Massachusetts Medical Center, where thousands of patients have been helped with chronic pain and stress-related medical disorders. The results are impressive. Patients who complete the eight-week course have both physical and psychological symptom reduction that lasts over time. People who come to the clinic with panic disorders have a dramatic drop in anxiety and panic levels; the reduction persists for at least three years. Even the patients' view of the world and their relationship to the world change.

For insurance companies to be giving medical reimbursement for learning to meditate, there must be more to it than gurus and mystical experiences, and there is. Jon Kabat-Zinn, the founder and Director of the Stress Reduction Clinic at the University of Massachusetts Medical Center, suggests, "One way to look at meditation is as a kind of intrapsychic technology that's been developed over a couple of thousand years by traditions that know a lot about the mind/body connection."

The scientific evidence is growing that good things happen in the body, mind, and spirit with regular meditation. Conversely, mystic Thomas Merton warned of the dangers that come from not allowing into our lives the "interior solitude" that comes in meditation. He said, "When society is made up of men who know no interior solitude, it can no longer be held together by love; and consequently it is held together by a violent and abusive authority." Sometimes we become our own "violent and abusive authority" by not making space in our lives for meditation.

Tibetan meditation master Sogyal Rinpoche says the real miracle of meditation is that it "is a subtle transformation, and this transformation happens not only in your mind and your emotions, but also in your body." Buddhist teacher Joseph Goldstein has found that "what happens as we practice [meditation] is that we bring the attention back and become a little more accepting of what's going on. When we do this, quite an amazing thing happens. We find that we're less driven, in meditation and in our lives, by the forces of denial and addiction."

The gifts of meditation are what the *Tao Te Ching* describes as the "greatest treasures."

Simplicity, patience, compassion.
These three are your greatest treasures.
Simple in action and in thoughts,
you return to the source of being.

Patient with both friends and enemies,
you accord with the way things are.
Compassionate toward yourself,
you reconcile all beings in the world.

How does this happen? How does meditation create such powerful effects? No one knows for sure, but people have some ideas. One theory is that meditation stops the production of stress-related hormones long enough for the body to repair and rejuvenate itself. Meditation may be such a powerful "pause that refreshes" in part because a physiological state is produced that is diametrically opposed to the physiological state created by anxiety and anger. When a person is meditating, heart, respiration, and metabolic rates decrease, and blood lactate levels drop. High levels of any of these measures are associated with anxiety and tension. Also, some glands produce hormones that lead to a state of well-being. When we meditate, the brain produces those hormones, called endorphins, which are natural opiates. A shot of endorphins from the brain can make us feel well and zestful for the rest of the day.

Another way meditation works is that it trains the mind to stop chattering so much. We have 60,000 thoughts a day. Kabat-Zinn observes, "Most people don't realize that the mind constantly chatters. And yet that chatter winds up being the force that drives us much of the day, in terms of what we do, what we react to, and how we feel. Meditation is a way of looking deeply into the chatter of the mind and body and becoming more aware of its patterns. By observing it, you free yourself from much of it. And the chatter will calm down."

The many benefits of meditation do not come without a cost. The cost is commitment to the task. The benefits listed above were reported by people who described themselves as frequent meditators. It requires disciplined practice, sometimes weeks or months, to see appreciable results. A commitment to meditation means setting aside time every day of your life for only meditation. Patience and persistence are necessary. Time spent relaxing or resting does not count and will not serve as a substitute. But the discipline doesn't have to be a boring burden. When you meditate, you are getting to know your mind and body intimately and learning the empowering possibilities of both. How could that possibly be boring? Approach it with a sense of discovery and you will be continually rewarded by the process. Sogyal Rinpoche advises, "In one sense meditation is an art, and you should bring to it an artist's delight and fertility of invention. Become as resourceful in inspiring yourself to enter your own peace as you are at being neurotic and competitive in the world."

Meditation is a stilling of the mind as well as the body. Both effects are required. It is a surrendering, for a few minutes twice a day, of our egos, our need to be doing, proving, pleasing. As Dom Laurence Freeman, a Benedictine monk dedicated to spreading the understanding of meditation in the Christian community, explains, "Meditation is the exercise, or, if you wish, the lack of exercise, the 'minus' exercise which repeatedly makes you acquainted with that secret emptiness, the apparent vacuum which is then irresistibly filled with the abundance of your life, of existence, of the whole life, of the whole universe, the power of the sun, of love, the importance of the atom."

Meditation is a commitment to humility and poverty of desire for a precious period of time each day. Making a commitment to sit still for twenty to thirty minutes once in the morning and once in the evening every day is very simple and extremely difficult. I encourage you to learn to meditate and to do whatever it takes to do so. For me, that means getting up earlier in the morning. It also means a sacrifice in terms of work— a financial sacrifice—because I have to schedule time into my calendar to meditate. All my client appointments are in my book, and so is my meditation time, but it took me a while to do that. I have learned to honor meditation time as much as I would honor my appointments with anybody else. I make a little less money now, but my life has certainly not been diminished. On the contrary, I have been enriched immensely. Making money has become less important to me, and yet there always seems to be enough for what I want or need.

Once you have made the commitment to meditate, there are four basic elements that need to be in place. Dr. Herbert Benson, one of the first medical scientists in the United States to research the effects of meditation, found that the following four conditions are essential. They are:

1. *A quiet place,* where you will not be disturbed for the duration of the meditation. I can now meditate with some satisfactory results even on a noisy airplane, but it takes much training in silence to be able to stay with it when there are distracting noises. Even though meditating under such adverse conditions is possible, the quality of the meditation is not as great and the benefits, I think, are less.

2. *A comfortable position with spine erect.* You can sit cross-legged on a cushion on the floor, or in a chair. Keep your head level or chin slightly tipped down. My meditation teacher observes that students are thinking rather than meditating if their heads are tipped backward and that they are dozing when their heads lean a bit too far forward.

3. *A passive attitude.* This means taking an observing stance, not trying to make anything happen, not struggling, not evaluating your performance. Just being with the experience, however that experience goes.

4. *Choice of a word, object, or your breath to focus on.* Two different forms of focusing are given in the exercises below. The act of continually "resting" your attention on one place, whether it is a sound, an image, or a sensation, may be a large part of what produces the physiological benefits described previously.

Stimulants, including caffeine or drugs of any kind,

will impair or prevent the meditative process. If you are taking any kind of prescription drugs, check with your physician. The practice of meditation can sometimes reduce the amount of medication necessary to control your problem. Hypertension, thyroid condition, some diabetes, and glaucoma all have been shown to respond to meditation. Your dosage may have to be adjusted as your body responds to the powerful effects of meditation.

In addition to arranging for the appropriate setting, assuming correct posture, and avoiding chemical substances that interfere, you should follow the insistence of all traditions of meditation teaching upon "right living." Right living is summed up thus: "Abstain from all sinful, unwholesome actions, perform all pious, wholesome ones, purify the mind, this is the teaching of all enlightened ones." You may not feel "right living" is attainable by you, now or ever. So aim higher. These are goals to be aspired to and not requirements for meditation. But meditation will be more beneficial if the rest of your life is aimed towards health and wholeness. Paradoxically, meditation also makes aiming for those goals easier. If we practice enough, the small miracles of life we all experience every day become meditations: a smile, a flower, the changing light of the morning. This ancient poem describes how it can be:

> Ten thousand flowers in spring, the moon in
>   autumn,
> a cool breeze in summer, snow in winter.

If your mind isn't clouded by unnecessary things,
this is the best season of your life.
—Wu-Men

There are many techniques of meditation. Two very ancient and simple ones are given in the following exercises.

Exercise: Meditation With a Mantra

Meditation with a mantra, or word/phrase, is very common. "Mantra" is a Sanskrit term meaning a "formula" of prayer or "one little word." The mantra word may be one that has a universal meaning or a particular history. "Om" (with a long "O") means God or "the One." Maranatha (said as four distinct syllables of equal length—Ma-Ra-Na-Tha) is an ancient Aramaic word/phrase meaning "Come, Lord" or "The Lord Comes." It is the mantra suggested by Christian teachers of meditation, such as the Benedictine monks John Main and Laurence Freeman. "Shalom," meaning peace, or secular words such as "one" or "peace" can be used. The mantra serves as a focal point or anchor to return to again and again as the mind drifts away.

The steps for meditating begin with sitting comfortably and upright on a chair or on a cushion on the floor. The important thing is to have the spine erect and to position yourself in an alert manner.

The next step is to be still. This means not wiggling,

scratching, or moving once the meditation time begins. Being still plays a large role in relinquishing the ego's control. Commitment to the goal of surrendering to stillness overrides the desires of the "I," including "I want to scratch/move."

Close your eyes gently and begin saying your word or mantra silently the entire period of the meditation. Listen to it as you say it. Say it gently but continuously. When you find your mind has wandered into thinking, remembering, daydreaming, planning, or any of those other mental activities that the mind is so easily drawn into, gently return to saying your mantra. Do not imagine or think anything, spiritual or otherwise. If great ideas come during the meditation, let them go and return to your mantra. That is the discipline. Relinquishing all wants, desires, clinging, for these few minutes.

Again, meditate each day, in the morning and in the afternoon or evening for twenty to thirty minutes.

Another form of meditation, perhaps even older than meditation using a mantra, is meditation that consists of focusing on the breath. This form of practice is called Vipassana, Mindfulness, or Insight Meditation. Insight results from the process of repeatedly being mindful of the moment.

Exercise: Insight Meditation

Vipassana meditation begins by focusing on a very

simple process that is always with us—breathing. Assume any sitting posture that is comfortable to you, keeping your back reasonably straight, without being stiff or strained. If you are in a cramped or bent-over position, you will more quickly become uncomfortable. Sit in a chair if you like. The important thing is to move as little as possible, at the very least not very often. Your eyes should be closed or almost closed.

There are several different ways to practice awareness of the breath. One way is to put your attention on the movement of your belly as you breathe. When you breathe in, the abdomen naturally rises or extends, and when you breathe out, it falls. Keep your attention on the movement of the abdomen, not imagining, not visualizing anything, just experiencing the sensation of the movement. Don't control or force the breath in any way; merely stay attentive to the rising, falling movement of the abdomen.

A second way is to be aware of the breath as it goes in and out of the nostrils, keeping the attention in the area around the outer rim of the nostrils or in the small triangle on the upper lip where the breath moves in and out. Simply be aware of the in and out of your breath, the subtle sensation as it passes over the upper lip or in and out of the nostrils. It might be helpful in the beginning to make mental notes either of "rising, falling" or "in, out." This aids in keeping the mind on the object. Remember, it is not a breathing exercise. It is the beginning exercise in mindfulness. When your mind wanders, just bring it back to focusing on the breath. Do this twenty to thirty minutes.

Start meditating with discipline. In time, you will find that you long for meditation as naturally as you long for water, food, or rest. It is all these for your spirit—water, food, rest—and much more. Meditation, like anything else, won't fix everything that's wrong with you, but it fixes a great deal. Do it if you can. Please.

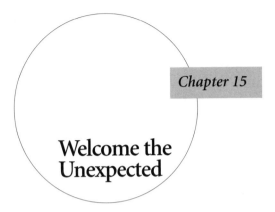

Chapter 15

Welcome the Unexpected

"The Master gives himself up
to whatever the moment brings."
—*Lao-tzu*

I consider everything we experience as an opportunity for enlightenment. To enlighten is "to put light into, make luminous, to remove dimness or blindness, to supply with intellectual light, to impart knowledge or wisdom, to instruct, inform, remove one's ignorance of something, to revive, exhilarate." It's a good thing to have happen to you, enlightenment is. Scott Peck, psychiatrist and author, says, "We cannot lose once we realize that everything that happens to us has been designed to teach us holiness."

I welcome what I feel in my body, be it illness, pain, or pleasure, because I am sure to end up knowing something unknown to me before. Pain, like a boil, may be the infection under the surface. When it comes to a head, it hurts, but the eruption is part of the process of healing.

Welcoming the unexpected is like unwrapping a surprise ball. When I was a child, a surprise ball was a highly prized party favor. It was made from a tightly wound one-inch-wide strips of colored crepe paper. The outside had a painted face, a jack-o-lantern, clown, or animal. When I unwound it, I uncovered tiny surprizes: a balloon, a whistle, a tiny plastic doll, a miniature puzzle. The trinkets were insignificant, but the finding, the discovery, the unwrapping of the mystery was the real prize. Not knowing what would be revealed but expecting something created a readiness for discovery. I was never disappointed in a surprise ball. There was always something waiting to be found inside.

Annie Dillard understands about surprise balls, the unexpected, and pennies. I like how she tells about them: "When I was six or seven years old, growing up in Pittsburgh, I used to take a precious penny of my own and hide it for someone else to find. It was a curious compulsion; sadly, I've never been seized by it since. For some reason, I always "hid" the penny along the same stretch of sidewalk up the street. I would cradle it at the root of a Sycamore, say, or in a hole left by a chipped-off piece of sidewalk. Then I would take a piece of chalk, and, starting at either end of the block, draw huge arrows leading up to the penny from both directions. After I learned to write I labeled the arrows: *surprise ahead* or *money this way*. I was greatly excited, during all this arrow-drawing, at the thought of the first lucky passer-by who would receive in this way, regardless of merit, a free gift from the universe. But I never lurked about. I would go straight home and not give the matter another thought, until, some months later, I would be gripped again by the impulse to hide another penny. … There are lots of things to see, unwrapped gifts and free surprises. The world is fairly studded and strewn with pennies cast broadside from a generous hand. … It is dire poverty indeed when a man is so malnourished and fatigued that he won't stoop to pick up a penny. But if you cultivate a healthy poverty and simplicity, so that finding a penny will literally make your day, then, since the world is in fact planted in pennies, you have with your poverty bought a lifetime of days. It is that simple. What you see is what you get."

By welcoming the unexpected, you learn to see the treasures in all you encounter—in your body, in your illness and wellness, in your life. I had a client who had suffered since childhood with what was finally diagnosed as rheumatoid arthritis. Her health improved rapidly and dramatically once she began doing the work to recover her body. Then one day her right knee suddenly swelled. "I've been so good!" she lamented. "I've been meditating, exercising, eating right. I don't understand it." She wept in defeat.

When her tears subsided, I asked her to tell her knee how she felt. "I don't understand you! You hurt me, and I don't know why. I never know what to expect of you." I asked if there was anyone else she could say those words to. "My dad!" she said with amazement. She then began an imaginary dialogue with her alcoholic father, expressing long-forgotten hurt and anger. The next morning, the swelling was gone from her knee. Her doctor's tests that day showed that her "sed rate" in her blood was normal for the first time in fifteen years, meaning there was no sign of inflammation. This woman had picked up the penny and found a treasure.

The unconscious often directs us to the pennies. The body is one way the unconscious—what we are unaware of—expresses itself. Different body postures express unconscious feelings and defenses. Illness and pain can do the same. My client's swollen knee was directing her to an unhealed wound in her psyche. The body can point the way if we trust it to guide us. It has an inner knowing that can be trusted.

In saying this, I am *not* claiming that only our minds cause physical illness. That is simply not true and implies an unfair indictment of anyone who gets sick. It is a belief in "disembodied spiritualism" that is as unrealistic as "mindless materialism," which implies there is nothing happening in the body that

cannot be explained or understood as a physical process. What I am saying is that emotional pain does play a role in physical illness and needs to be honored and acknowledged.

Richard knew his leg was broken even before

he felt the blast of pain or saw the splintered bones sticking through his skin. Instantly he relaxed. He knew the right thing had happened. "Never once did I regret the accident," Richard said as he settled his 6'5" frame on the sofa and arranged his left leg, which was still in a cast seven months after the accident. "I had to have this happen. I literally had to be crushed to be stopped. I was headed down a path that was wrong, and there's no way I could have stopped myself."

The accident happened when Richard was cleaning his pool. He's a very big man. When his right foot slipped, the whole weight of his 250-pound body fell on his left leg. It broke in five places, and some of the ankle bones were crushed. After six operations, the doctors tell him he's lucky he didn't lose his leg. Richard thinks he's lucky for more than that. He thinks he's fortunate the whole thing happened just the way it did.

"I was lucky that I had a portable phone by me. I called my wife in the house. She came running out and called 911. The emergency people were there in seven minutes. I had great doctors. Most of all, I am lucky—no, blessed—that I was forced to detour off of a crash course. I was driving myself so hard that I know something bad was going to happen to me before long. Something in my body was going to give out. I needed a long rest for my body and my mind. Money and deals had become my god. I lost sight of what really matters: my wife, my sons, my health, loving God. Yes, I'm very lucky. The moment this happened, I felt calm. At last, I could relax. My freefall had been halted. I have no 'if onlys' and feel blessed even if I walk with a limp or have some pain the rest of my life. If I do, I'll just see it as a needed reminder of how I was saved in the nick of time."

Clarissa Pinkola Estés defines intuition as a "divining instrument and like a crystal through which one can see with uncanny interior vision. It is like a wise old woman who is with you always, who tells you exactly what the matter is, who tells you exactly whether you need to go left or right." I think the body is a physical manifestation of that intuition. We are all born intuitive. What we lack is not intuition but the courage to act on what we intuit, what we know is true for us.

When a client tells me of some accident or illness, I ask, "What's really wrong?" What is usually wrong is not the cold or flu or sprained ankle. Those are the manifestations of what is indeed wrong. They are also the signposts pointing the way to the healing. Steven Levine, author of *Healing Into Life and Death*, believes, "Healing is what happens when we come to our edge, to the unexplored territory of mind and body, and take a single step beyond into the unknown, the space in which all growth occurs. Healing is discovery." Welcoming the unexpected is making room for discovery. Artist Agnes Martin, in her eighties and enjoying an active creative life, advises, "The adventurous state of mind is a high house. To enjoy life, the adventurous state of mind must be grasped and maintained.

The essential feature of adventure is that it is a going forward into unknown territory."

In working with the dying and people with life-threatening illness, Levine observed, "Among those who seemed to move toward healing, physical and psychological as well as spiritual, there seemed to be many who had a certain quality in common. They had a willingness, a kind of open relationship to the conditions they were experiencing, a certain nonresistance … a new willingness to take the teaching from whatever moment illness presented; the leading edge of life to be examined and participated in. These were the people who embraced their pain and fear, and met what had always been conditioned by fear and loathing with a new openness, and at times a new wonderment of life." Welcoming the unexpected is about embracing all of your life, including the pain.

A wise man once said, "This is not a perfect world, but it is a sacred world." The body is never perfect, but it is always sacred. Pain and pleasure will always coexist. If you expect perfection in your body, you will always feel betrayed. No matter how well-attuned you are to your body, it will change and deteriorate with age. The physical body, which holds our lives, will die. In that sense, our best friend, our body, brings about the ultimate betrayal—death. But the death of the body has little to do with how alive we can feel, except perhaps to remind us that each moment is precious and ought to be experienced as fully as possible. So don't deceive

yourself by looking for perfection—no illness, deformity, pain, brokenness—in your body. It's not going to
happen. It's not supposed to. Look instead for whatever
your body brings as an opportunity for enlightenment.
Learn to welcome the lessons, even if they are unexpected and painful. Welcome the communication.

To communicate is "to impart knowledge of; make
known; to give or interchange thoughts, feelings, information, or the like, by writing, speaking, etc."
Communication offers the possibility for understanding, be that between husband and wife, parent and
child, teacher and student, or mind and body. The following exercise can facilitate communication between
you and your body and help you be a little more open to
the unexpected.

Exercise: Let's Talk

When you have something "wrong" with your
body, a cold, a headache, a sprain, a break, or any illness,
enter a dialogue with the problem.

Imagine your problem, a headache, for example, as
a person. With paper and pen in hand, begin asking it
questions and record both the questions and answers.
If you prefer, you can tape record the dialogue. Just be
patient if no answers seem forthcoming. Your body
may need a little time to be convinced that you are
really interested in what it has to tell you, especially if
you have long neglected your body and ignored its

messages. This won't work if you rush or force it.

These are some possibilities for the dialogue:

☞ Tell the illness or injury how you feel about its being there.

☞ Tell it what problems it's causing you.

☞ Tell it what it's doing to you and how.

☞ Ask it why it's there.

☞ Ask what it wants you to know.

☞ Ask what it wants you to do.

☞ Ask if there is some way you can work out a plan so that you don't need the illness or injury.

☞ Acknowledge what you're learning from it.

☞ Thank it for trying to teach you.

☞ Acknowledge your part in making the teaching necessary.

☞ Thank it for what you are learning, for the opportunity to change and heal.

That last part of this exercise—expressing appreciation—may be difficult. But do it even if you do not really feel you mean it just yet. The words are important, and resistance begins to dissolve as we can acknowledge the gift in what is happening.

End the exercise with the Golden Light imaging. Get in a comfortable position and gently close your eyes. See a Golden Light emanating from a Divine Presence or just coming from somewhere outside yourself, and let it flow first into the part of you that is ill or hurting. Imagine it coming into that place with each inhalation and the pain going out with each exhalation. Breathe slowly and deeply. After a few moments, see or feel the warm Golden Light flowing into your pure center, the part of you that is well, whole, uninjured always. Let the Light flow in with each breath, connecting with your purity. As the Light touches and penetrates you, allow it to cleanse and purify all your wounds, pain, suffering, destructive emotions, and shame. Let yourself be dissolved into the Light, even if for only a moment. Rest in this renewing, restoring Light. As the Light fades, express your "thank you" and slowly open your eyes. Now go about your business of life, knowing you are now a little more welcoming of the unexpected and at peace in a body you have recovered and reclaimed.

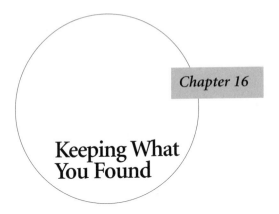

Chapter 16

Keeping What You Found

> "If you don't break your ropes while you're alive,
>   do you think ghosts will do it after?"
> *—Kabir*

Now that you have done and are doing the hard work of reowning and recovering your body, it only makes sense not to lose it again. How can you do that—keep what you have regained? First, make up your mind now that you won't ever live in a deadened, numb body again. Deciding that isn't actually too hard. Once you are out of the land of darkness and pain and living in the Light, there's not much appeal in going back again, even if there's some temptation to return to the familiar. We've all lived through some experience or time we would never want to relive. "I don't ever want to go through that again" is the refrain. "That" may be having preschool children, remodeling an old house, drinking to excess,

275

being obese, or raging in a marriage. Not living in your body is like that, a misery you could and did endure but never want to experience again.

So just being back in your own body will do some of the work of motivating you to stay there. But that's not enough. Make it a promise. "I won't live that way again!" The promise will stay in your memory even if the pain of living in a lost body fades. That's Step One. Step Two is to keep doing all the things that helped you to recover that aliveness. You won't have to put in all the time, effort, and anguish that you did at the beginning, but you *will* have to keep up a maintenance program. Recovering your body may have been like coming out of anesthesia. The unconscious sleep might have seemed preferable to the pain you first felt when your recovery began. Once the healing begins, though, you know you are so much better off that you wonder how you could have lived the way you were before. By making the exercises in this book a part of your life, you ensure that you don't go back.

To stay recovered means staying committed to conscious living, which begins with being conscious of your body. As you have worked the exercises in this book, your conscious awareness of your body sensations has increased. You know much more about when you are breathing and how. You know more about how you move, hold yourself, see, eat, feel sexual or angry. If you have had any bodywork, you've learned how and where you hold tension and what happens when you release it from a specific muscle group. You've seen how your tension mirrors your inflexibility and fear. You've had some practice in letting your body and your emotions change and have learned perhaps to be a bit more welcoming of what you didn't expect. If you've started meditating, all sorts of connections are being made between physical, mental, emotional, and spiritual spheres. Some you may be aware of already, and some may still be too subtle to be detected just yet. For all you've done, no matter how little or how much, congratulations! Every step counts and moves you more deeply into a recovered body, giving you aliveness that is your birthright.

Just don't quit! Without breath, we all die in a few short minutes. Without movement, our muscles atrophy. Without the nutrition appropriate for the body, it becomes ill, emaciated, or bloated with fat. We have to keep giving our bodies what they need. As I said in Chapter 1, *Alive and Well* is both a first aid book and an owner's manual. You've done the first-aid emergency work. Now do the maintenance exercises to keep your body in "good working order."

My recommendation is that you start again at the beginning of the book and work through it just as you did the first time, with inquisitiveness and trepidation. You won't be doing the same thing again, even when you do the same exercises. It's simply not possible. No one steps into the same river twice. That ancient saying applies here. The very first breath exercise will be different for you now that you have done so much work. Every exercise will be. You will make new discoveries and move to a different level of awareness and aliveness. Think of it as any experience you repeat: saying a prayer, jogging, making love, putting your child to bed at night, eating a bowl of cereal. It's never the same, even though you're going through basically the same motions. It's never the same because you're never the same. Let the exercises in this book become a part of how you live. Do them daily. Re-try the more difficult or least enjoyable ones.

My client Peter told me a story of how he had found great solace in eating mindfully. Peter had just learned that there were budget uncertainties at work. Many people were going to be laid off, and he might be one of them. This meant he was going to have to stop therapy for the time being in order to conserve money. That, combined with a relationship crisis, left him feeling shaky, sad, and frightened. "I was sitting there eating the second of my 85 cent blueberry muffins," he said. "Suddenly it hit me that this was my world. Just this muffin and me. I began to taste the soft, warm, sweetness of it, and I felt so nurtured and cared for, that this food was provided for me. I felt a great sense of relief and much less lonely."

Peter might have missed this awareness had he not already had some experience with eating mindfully. You never know which of these exercises you will draw on in times of pain or crisis. Like CPR or prayer, you want to have the knowledge and learned experience available when you need it. So practice the exercises over and over until you have a storehouse to draw from anytime you need recovering. Do these exercises until you know you live in your body and can stay in it no matter what's happening inside or outside of you. Repeating the exercises ensures that you will keep what you found—your recovered body and your aliveness. Make sure you do keep them. You deserve to feel that good. Your body is yours. You own it. Finally, for the effort you have made and will make in recovering your body, I thank you. We are all better off for your having done so.

Notes

"The body's a mirror of heaven…" *Rumi, p. 8.*

INTRODUCTION

The definitions of "recover" in the *Oxford English Dictionary* in Vol. XIII, p. 367.

"We replace 98 percent of every atom…," Deepak Chopra, in address on June 22-27, 1993.

"The body is a river…," Chopra, same address as above.

"I am a soul with a hundred thousand bodies…," Rumi, p. 84.

"Our beliefs, attitudes and basic positions toward life all shape the way we react…," Blair Justice, pp. 63-64.

The research by Drs. Trickett and Putnam is discussed in the article by Tori De Angelis, p. 1, 38.

For a discussion on posture and emotional suffering, see Kurtz and Prestera's *The Body Reveals.*

"energies of an addiction…," Marion Woodman, 1992, p. 26.

"It is not that there is no distinction between pure and impure…," Stephen Mitchell, *The Gospel According to Jesus*, p. 154.

Chapter 1: HOW TO USE THIS BOOK

"Living never wore one out so much…," Anäis Nin's quote is from *A Woman's Journal.*

Chapter 2: YOUR BODY KNOWS: MEMORIES, EXPERIENCE, AND REALITY

"Reality is perceived…," Sutras are Hindu teachings. "Sutra" is a sanskrit word meaning "thread." The small teachings are threaded together to give greater wisdom. "Vimalakirti sutras" are threads without blemish or impurity.

Stages of change were investigated by Prochaska, DiClemente, & Norcross, pp. 1102-1104.

Rubenfeld's definition of body memory, from Mirka Knaster, "Remembering...Through the Body," p. 47.

"Memory resides nowhere...," Knaster, p. 47.

"Memory is influenced...," is a quote from Ornstein in the article by Knaster, p. 47.

Research on how young toddlers may remember is discussed in the article by Daniel Goleman.

"So our memories, as exact, recorded fixed images...," *Massage Therapy Journal*, Winter 1994, p. 47.

Declarative and emotional memories are discussed by Joseph LeDoux in "Emotion, Memory and the Brain," June 1994, pp. 50-57.

Neurologist-physician Oliver Sacks' story is told in his interview in *Profile Magazine*, pp. 39-41. The quote is from p. 41.

Dr. Bessel van der Kolk discussed his theory of traumatic memories and their recovery in two films, *Trauma and Memory I—The Dissociative Defense* and *Trauma and Memory II—The Intrusive Past*, 1993.

Pictures of the brain remembering, a discussion of research by Marcus Raichle & Larry R. Squire, is in the article by Hilts, in *The New York Times*, November 11, 1991.

"Hit a tripwire...," Diane Ackerman, p. 5.

"Smell is a potent wizard...," Ackerman, p. 3.

"a whiff of the type of paste," Ackerman, pp.17-18.

"We never really forget anything...," Frederick Buechner, author, Presbyterian minister, p. 70.

Eileen Franklin's example of a flashback being triggered by a visual memory, p. 6.

"I do believe that words hang...," interview with Maya Angelou by C. J. Houtchens, p. 5.

Lynn Redgrave's story is from her play, *Shakespeare for My Father*, which is in press.

The findings on disconnection of girls from themselves as they enter adolescence is discussed in the *Final Report* on the Harvard Project on Women's Psychology and Girls' Development.

"It's not a matter of dancing on mechanical legs...," Marion Woodman, 1993, p. 29.

For more information on dissociation and denial, see Cornell and Olio, pp. 131-143.

"a primitive and desperate unconscious method of coping...," Laughlin, p. 57.

"this can't be happening to me...," Riekur and Carmen, p. 365.

"numb and dumb" are discussed by Cornell and Olio, p. 135.

"Contact-satisfaction-withdrawal cycle" from Smith, *The Body in Psychotherapy*, p. 36.

Anxiety drugs and the risks discussed in *Consumer Reports*, p. 20.

Chapter 3: BODYWORK: What it is, Why do it, Whom to chose

"A body who has lived a long time accumulates debris. It cannot be avoided...," Estés, p. 364.

To read more about pioneers in the early part of this century who saw the necessity of working with the body as well as the psyche, see Smith, Chapter 1, "The Tradition of the Body in Psychotherapy," pp. 3-28.

The history of bodywork is discussed by Juhan, pp. xx-xxii.

"Bodywork was critically important to me...," Marilyn Van Derbur, private correspondence, Dec, 1992.

An explanation of how touch can provide a sensorimotor education is given by Juhan, p. xxix.

"I am convinced that for every physical non-yielding condition...," Dr. Milton Trager in Juhan, p. xxv.

Bodyworker as a "diplomatic intermediary...they administer is self-awareness," Juhan, p. xxix.

Effects of touch on premature babies is discussed by Ackerman, pp. 71-80.

Dr. Saul Schanberg is quoted in Ackerman, pp. 77-78.

"But when we lose touch…," Ackerman, p. 82.

Non-psychotherapeutic bodywork and psychotherapy which involves bodywork are discussed by Smith, pp. 148-153.

"If the therapist makes you feel worthless, find another therapist…," Quinnart.

Bodywork "can help us recall that we are living, growing systems…," Juhan, p. xxx.

"By their deeds…," a paraphrasing of Matthew 7:20, which reads: "Therefore by their fruits you will know them."

Chapter 4: START BREATHING

"I will sing to you at every moment; I will praise you with every breath." Psalm 104, "The Book of Psalms," in *The Enlightened Heart*, p. 8.

"There's not a single neurotic…," Smith, p. 121.

"The fact is that we are painters…," Van Gogh is quoted by Louise Bourgeois in the notes from her exhibit at the Corcoran.

"The fact is…," Dillard, p. 240.

For more information on the effect on breathing from trauma in the birthing process or during gestation, see Verny & Kelly, *The Secret Life of the Unborn Child*.

For more information on pranayama and its purpose, see Chopra, *Perfect Health*, pp. 298, 322.

Right brain/left brain dialogue is explained by Chopra, same source, pp. 298-299.

Chapter 5: GET MOVING

"How infinite in faculty, in form, and moving!" is from William Shakespeare's *Hamlet*, p. 1062.

Two-thirds of Americans do no kind of vigorous exercise on a regular basis, says Paul Z. Siegel, M.D., in an interview in *Bottom Line Newsletter*, April 15, 1992.

"For many of us, the body is a feared enemy…," Gabrielle Roth, *Maps to Ecstasy*, pp. 30-31.

"We let our bodies go the way of our fears…," Dillard, p. 90.

"…only 30 minutes of aerobic exercise…," Jöhnsgard, pp. 279-280.

"Angels find it easier…," Caroline Myss said this in her workshop at the Noetic Sciences Annual Conference, 1993.

"Whether one is an experienced athlete or a beginner…," Jöhnsgard, p. 287.

"Movement is the medium…," Gabrielle Roth, 1991, p. 23.

"mild to moderate exercise produces…," Jöhnsgard, p. 197.

The exercise *Silly Moving* was created by Trudi Schoop, p. 86.

The exercise *Split Bodies* was also designed by Schoop, pp. 108-109.

Gabrielle Roth's approach to dancing the "sacred rhythms" is described in her book *Maps to Ecstasy*, pp. 31-34.

When we watch a seventy-year-old hand…," Emile Da'oud is quoted by Stephen Mitchell in his translation of the *Tao Te Ching*, pp. 88-89.

Chapter 6: GET GROUNDED

"I wonder if I shall fall…," Lewis Carroll, p. 5.

Definition of grounding is in *The American Heritage Dictionary of the English Language*.

The relationship between emotions and how we relate to the ground is discussed by Kurtz and Prestera, p. 38.

"Chatter" is explained by Kurtz and Prestera, pp. 37-38.

"As we go through our work…," Joseph Goldstein, *Living Wisdom*, p. 3.

"A priest, in advancing and returning, has an accurate comprehension of what he does…," Needleman, pp. 152-153.

"Without the protective shell…," Jöhnsgard, p, 54.

Deepak Chopra talked about speeded-up biological clocks in his address at the Noetic Sciences Conference.

Tao Te Ching, #64, translated by Stephen Mitchell.

Chapter 7: START OBSERVING

"The moment you settle down…," Katsuki Sekida, p. 228.

"From a meditative perspective…," Jon Kabat-Zinn, p. 122.

Kabat-Zinn's story of the sweating woman and his quote, p. 122.

"It's all a matter of keeping my eyes open…," Dillard, p. 17.

Chapter 8: LET IT CHANGE

The only thing that makes life possible…," Ursula K. LeGuin's quote is from *A Woman's Journal*.

"This existence of ours is as transient as autumn clouds…," Sogyal Rinpoche, p. 25.

"Impermanence is like some of the people we meet in life…," Sogyal Rinpoche, p. 25.

"Not only does something come if you wait…," Dillard, p. 259.

"We are terrified of letting go…," Sogyal Rinpoche, p. 33.

Chapter 9: APPRECIATE THE VEHICLE

"And all must love the human form…," Blake, p. 59.

"I ran into a rabbi…," Roth in *Maps to Ecstasy*, p. 30.

"What is needed for the body…," Andrew Harvey said this in an interview with Rose Solari for *Common Boundary* magazine, p. 36.

"Some say the body holds…," McCauley.

"Angst about the body robs a woman…," Estés, p. 204.

"The issue is not what shape, what size…," Estés, p. 208.

"The infant cries…," Mitchell, *The Gospel According to Jesus*, p. 215.

"I didn't look…," Monica Seles was interviewed by Robin Flynn, *The New York Times*, Friday, August 27, 1993, pp. B9-B10, and quoted in *The Houston Post*, Thursday, August 26, 1993, pp. C1-C11.

Chapter 10: WATCH YOUR EYES

"In our minds…," from an interview with artist Agnes Martin.

"The eye is the lamp of the body…," Mitchell, *The Gospel According to Jesus*, p. 181.

"At that time I still wanted to use my eyes…," Lusseyran, pp. 16ff.

Chapter 11: EAT MINDFULLY

"80 million people in this country are dieting…," Hirschmann & Munter, p. 9.

The diet industry is a $12 billion a year business, Hirschmann & Munter, p. 3.

Zen story and discussion of mindful eating, Goldstein, *The Experience of Insight*, p. 50.

The exercise *Body Check/Hunger Check* is by Geneen Roth, pp. 11-12.

"When you fast…," Matthew 6:16-18.

Chapter 12: DIRECT THE ANGER

Just as the physical pain tells us…," Harriet Goldhor Lerner, p. 1.

"Anger is the firestorm…," Cameron, p. 62.

"A temperamentally angry man…," Thomas Merton, pp. 23-24.

Research done at the University of British Columbia, reported in Marilyn Elias, "Expressing anger varies for two sexes," *The Houston Post*, August 28, 1993, p. F3.

Research on women's anger reported in "Women get angry, express it, too," *The Houston Post*, November 14, 1993, p. A-12.

The relationship between awareness and raging is discussed by

Hightower, pp. 15-33.

"The occurrence of an evil thought…," Seiki, p. 35.

Ten Anger Management Exercises are from Hightower.

Turn Off the Road to Anger exercise, Jean Deschener, pp. 156-157.

John Coon is the Director of The Yoga Center of Houston.

The exercise *Get Off My Back* is by Alexander Lowen & Leslie Lowen, p. 86.

The *No! No! No!* exercise is also from Lowen and Lowen, pp. 108-109.

Chapter 13: REOWN YOUR SEXUALITY

"Sex is difficult…," Rilke, pp. 50-51.

"I've had all the out-of-body experiences…," Harvey in his interview with Rose Solari, p. 36.

"We don't just kiss…," Ackerman, p. 112.

The case studies reported by Doctors Gizzi and Gitler and the relationship between heart attacks and bigamy are discussed by Larry Dossey, pp. 36-37.

Chapter 14: MEDITATE DAILY

"There are seconds…," F. Dostoevski, p. 586.

The benefits for frequent meditators are discussed by Beauchamp-Turner and Levinson, pp. 123-129.

Jon Kabat-Zinn and the Stress Reduction Clinic are discussed in Bill Moyers, *Healing and the Mind.* "One way to look at meditation…," p. 116.

"When society is made up…," Thomas Merton, pp. 23-24.

"a subtle transformation…," Sogyal Rinpoche, p. 80.

What happens as we practice…," Joseph Goldstein, Living Wisdom, p. 3.

"Simplicity, patience, compassion…," *Tao Te Ching*, Mitchell, #67.

"Meditation produces a physiological state…," Herbert Benson's chapter on meditation is in Nucho, p. 81.

"60,000 thoughts a day…," Deepak Chopak cited this figure in his address to the Noetic Sciences Conference, 1993.

"Meditation is truly the 'pause that refreshes,'" concluded Ani Nucho, p. 82.

"Most people don't realize…," Kabat-Zinn, p. 115.

"In one sense meditation is an art…," Sogyal Rinpoche, p. 80.

"Meditation is the exercise…," Dom Laurence Freeman, p. ix.

Four essentials of meditation are discussed by Benson in Nucho, p. 78.

Right living means to "Abstain from all sinful, unwholesome actions, perform all pious wholesome ones…," is from Chiu-Nan's chapter in Nucho, p. 91.

"Ten thousand flowers in spring…," Wu-Men, in *The Enlightened Heart*, p. 47.

Meaning of a Mantra is explained by Freeman, p. 6.

The instruction on insight meditation is given by Joseph Goldstein in *The Experience of Insight*, pp. 4-5.

Chapter 15: WELCOME THE UNEXPECTED

The Master gives himself up…," Lao-tzu in Mitchell's *The Gospels According to Jesus*, p. 272.

The definition of enlighten is from the *Oxford English Dictionary*, p. 268.

"We cannot lose…," Scott Peck said this in a talk in Houston for The Hospice at the Texas Medical Center, Nov. 10, 1992.

"When I was six or seven years old…," Dillard, pp. 14-15.

Dr. David Spiegel discussed disembodied spiritualism in his talk, "Does Living Better Mean Living Longer? Effects of Supportive Group Therapy on Cancer Patients." Lecture presented at Society of Behavioral Medicine Annual Meeting, San Francisco, March 12, 1993.

"A divining instrument…," Estés, p. 74.

"Healing is what happens…," Levine, *Healing Into Life and Death*, p. 4.

"The adventurous state of mind…," Agnes Martin.

"Among those who seemed to move toward healing…," Levine, pp. 8-9.

Definition of "communicate" is from *The Random House Dictionary of the English Language*, p. 298.

Chapter 16: KEEPING WHAT YOU FOUND

"If your don't break your ropes…," Bly, 1971, 1977.

References

Ackerman, D. 1991. *A Natural History of the Senses.* New York: Vintage Books.

American Heritage Dictionary of the English Language. 1981. Ed. by William Morris. Houghton Mifflin, Boston.

A Woman's Journal. 1985. Phildelphia: Running Press.

Beauchamp-Turner, D.L., & Levinson, D.M. 1992. Effects of Meditation on Stress, Health, and Affect. *Medical Journal of Psychotherapy 5,* pp. 123-129.

Blake W. 1989. The Divine Image. *The Complete Prose and Poetry of William Blake.* Ed. by Geoffrey Keynes. London: The Nonesuch Press, p. 59.

Bourgeois, Louise. *The Locus of Memory, Works 1982-1993.* Notes from the exhibit at the Corcoran Gallery of Art, Washington, D.C. September 24, 1994-January 8, 1995.

Buechner, F. 1982. *The Sacred Journey.* New York: Walker and Co.

Cameron, J. 1992. *The Artist's Way: A Spiritual Path to Higher Creativity.* New York: Jeremy P. Tarcher/Perigee.

Carroll, L. 1866. *Alice's Adventures in Wonderland.* New York: William Morris.

Chopra, D. 1991. *Perfect Health.* New York: Harmony Books.

Chopra, D. June 22-27, 1993. Address at "The Heart of Healing" Noetic Science Conference, Arlington, Virginia. Collins, C. S. February 1994.

Consumer Reports. January 1993. "High Anxiety," pp. 19-24.

Cornell, W.F., & Olio, K.A. July 1992. Consequences of Childhood Bodily Abuse: A Clinical Model for Affective Interventions. *Transactional Analysis Journal 22*(3), pp. 131-143.

De Angelis, T. April 1995. New threat associated with child abuse. *The APA Monitor,* 26(4), pp. 1, 38.

Deschener, J. 1984. *The Hitting Habit: Anger Control for Battering Couples.* New York: The Free Press, pp. 156-157.

Dillard, A. 1988. *Pilgrim at Tinker Creek.* New York: Harper Perennial.

Dossey, L. 1991. *Meaning and Medicine.* New York: Bantam.

Dostoevski, F. 1953. *The Devils.* Harmondsworth, England: Penguin.

Elias, M. August 28, 1993. Expressing anger varies for two sexes. *The Houston Post*, p. F3.

Estés, C.P. 1992. *Women Who Run with the Wolves*. New York: Ballantine Books.

Franklin, E. 1991. *The Sins of the Father*. New York: Crown Publishers Inc.

Freeman, L. 1986. *Light Within: The Inner Path of Meditation*. New York: Crossroad Publishing Company.

Gilligan, C., Rogers, A., Geismar, K., Noel, N., O'Neill, K., & Thompson, H. 1993. Strengthening healthy resistance and courage in girls: A prevention project and a developmental study. *Final Report* presented to the Lilly Endowment. Unpublished manuscript of the Harvard Project on Women's Psychology and Girls' Development.

Goldstein, J. 1987. *The Experience of Insight*. Boston: Shambhala.

Goldstein, J. Fall 1992. Living Wisdom. *Insight Meditation Society (IMS) Newsletter*, p.3.

Goleman, D. April 4, 1993. Studying the secrets of childhood memory. *The New York Times*, p. B5,B8.

Harvey, A. 1988. *Love's Fire: Recreations of Rumi*. Ithaca, New York: Meeramma, p. 8.

Harvey, A. September/October 1994. "On divine responsibility." Interview by R. Solari. *Common Boundary*, pp. 32-37.

Hightower, N. March 1989. Working with Rageful and Violent Patients in Group Psychotherapy. *Houston Group Psychotherapy Journal* 3(1), pp. 15-33.

Hilts, P.J. November 11, 1991. Photos show mind recalling a word. *The New York Times,* p A1.

Hirschmann, J.R., & Munter, C.H. 1988. *Overcoming Overeating*. New York: Fawcett Columbine.

Houtchens, C.J. October 8-10, 1993. The word according to Maya Angelou. *USA WEEKEND*.

Jöhnsgard, K.W. 1989. *The Exercise Prescription for Depression and Anxiety*. New York: Plenum Press.

Juhan, Deane. 1987. *Job's Body*. Barrytown, New York: Station Hill Press.

Justice, B. 1988. *Who Gets Sick*. Los Angeles: Jeremy P. Tarcher, pp. 63-64.

Justice, R., & Justice, B. 1990. Of soul-mending and mountain climbing: Leading a four-day group therapy experience. *The Journal of the Houston Group Psychotherapy Society 4*(1), pp. 7-28.

Kabat-Zinn, J. 1993. Meditation. *In Healing and the Mind*. Ed. by Bill Moyers. New York: Doubleday.

Kabir. 1977. In Robert Bly's *The Kabir Book*. Beacon Press.

Knaster, M. Winter 1994. "Remembering....through the body." *Massage Therapy Journal*, pp. 46-59.

Kurtz, R., & Prestera, H. 1984. *The Body Reveals*. New York: Harper Collins.

Lambert, M.J. 1989. The individual therapist's contribution to psychotherapy process and outcome. *Clinical Psychology Review 9*, pp. 469-85.

LeDoux, J. June 1994. Emotion, memory, and the brain. *Scientific American*, pp. 50-57.

Lerner, H.G. 1985. *The Dance of Anger*. New York: Harper & Row, p. 1.

Levine, S. 1987. *Healing into Life and Death*. New York: Anchor Press/Doubleday.

Lowen, A., & Lowen, L. 1977. *The Way to Vibrant Health: A Manual of Bioenergetic Exercises*. New York: Harper & Row.

Jacques Lusseyran. 1963. *And There Was Light*. Elizabeth R. Cameron, Trans. Boston, Massachusetts: Little, Brown and Co.

Martin, A. 1993. *Gallery Notes* from exhibit at the Contemporary Arts Museum, Houston, Texas.

McCauley, G. 1992. *On the Mend*. No Bright Shield. Bronx, New York: Something More Publications.

Merton, T. 1958. *Thoughts in Solitude*. New York: The Noonday Press/Farrar, Strauss, & Giroux, p.13.

Mitchell, S. 1989. *The Enlightened Heart: An Anthology of Sacred Poetry*. New York: Harper and Row.

Mitchell, S. 1993. *The Gospel According to Jesus*. New York: Harper Perennial.

Mitchell, S. 1988. *Tao Te Ching*. New York: Harper & Row.

Myss, C. June 22-27, 1993. Workshop at The Heart of Healing, Noetic Science Conference, Arlington, Virginia.

Napier, N. May/June 1992. In S. C. Roberts, Multiple Realities. *Common Boundary*, p. 29.

Needleman, J. 1975. *A Sense of the Cosmos*. New York: Doubleday.

Nucho, A.O. 1988. *Stress Management: The Quest for Zest.* Spring-
field, Illinois: Charles C. Thomas Publisher.

Oxford English Dictionary. 1989. R. W. Burchfield (Ed.). Oxford:
Clarendon Press. Vol. XIII, p. 367.

Peck, S. November 10, 1992. Growing up. *Hospice Talk.* Publication
of the Texas Medical Center.

Prochaska, J.O., DiClemente, C.C., & Norcross, J.C. September
1992. In search of how people change: Applications to addic
tive behaviors. *American Psychologist* 47(9), pp.1102-1104.

Quinnart, P. 1982. *The Troubled People Book.* New York: The
Continuum Publishing Company.

Random House Dictionary of the English Language. 1966. J. Stein,
(Ed.). New York: Random House.

Redgrave, L. 1994. *Shakespeare For My Father.* (In press.)

Riekur, P., & Carmen, E. 1986. The victim-to-patient process: The
disconfirmation and transformation of abuse. *American
Journal of Orthopsychiatry 56*, pp.360-370.

Rilke, R. M. 1993. *Letters to a Young Poet.* Trans. by S. Mitchell.
Boston: Shambhala.

Roberts, W. August 7, 1993. Hospital to write novel prescription.
Interview by Debra Beachy. *Houston Chronicle*, pp. 1D, 3D.

Roth, Gabrielle. 1989. *Maps to Ecstasy: Teachings of an Urban
Shaman.* San Rafael, California: New World Library.

Roth, Geneen. 1986. *Breaking Free from Compulsive Eating.* New
York: North American Library.

Sacks, O. February 1994. "Doctor of the Soul." Interview by C. S.
Collins in *Profiles* (The Magazine of Continental Airlines), pp.
39-41.

Schoop, T., with Mitchell, P. 1974. *Won't You Join the Dance?* Palo
Alto, California: Mayfield Publishing Company.

Sekida, K. 1985. *Zen Training: Methods and Philosophy.* New York:
Weatherhill.

Seles, M. Interviewed by Robin Flynn in *The New York Times,*
August 27, 1993, pp. B9-B10. Also quoted in *The Houston Post,*
August 26, 1993, pp. C1, C11.

Shakespeare, William. 1942. The Tragedy of Hamlet, Prince of
Denmark. In *The Complete Plays and Poems of William
Shakespeare.* Ed. by William Allan Neilson and Charles
Jarvis Hill. Cambridge, Massachusetts: Houghton Mifflin Co.

Siegel, P.Z. April 15, 1992. Behavioral Risk Factor Surveillance Surveys for the Centers for Disease Control and Prevention. *Bottom Line Personals.*

Smith, E.W.L. 1985. *The Body in Psychotherapy.* Jefferson, North Carolina: McFarland and Co.

Sogyal, R. 1992. *The Tibetan Book of Living and Dying.* Editors: P. Gaffney and A. Harvey. San Francisco: Harper San Francisco.

Spiegel, D.M. March 12, 1993. Does living better mean living longer? Group therapy on cancer patients. Lecture presented at Society of Behavioral Medicine Annual Meeting, San Francisco.

Woodman, M. 1993. *Leaving My Father's House.* Boston: Shambhala.

Woodman, M. July/August 1992. In Her Own Voice. Interview by A.A. Simpkinson, *Common Boundary,* pp.22-29.

Women get angry and express it, too. November 14, 1993. *The Houston Post,* p. A-12.

Van Derbur, M. December 1992. Private correspondence.

Van der Kolk, Bessel. 1993. *Trauma and Memory I—The Dissociative Defense; Trauma and Memory II—The Intrusive Past.* Ukiah, California: Cavalcade Productions.

Verny, T., & Kelly, J. 1981. *The Secret Life of the Unborn Child.* New York: Summit Books.

Copyright Acknowledgements

I am grateful to the following for permission to reprint brief passages from the copyrighted works named:

The Free Press, a Division of Simon & Schuster Inc. from *The Hitting Habit: Anger Control for Battering Couples* by Jeanne P. Deschner. Copyright © 1984 by The Free Press.

HarperCollins from *Pilgrim At Tinker Creek* by Annie Dillard. Copyright © 1974 by Annie Dillard.

Newton Hightower from Working with Rageful and Violent Patients in Group Psychotherapy, *Houston Group Psychotherapy Journal* 3,(1), pp. 15-33. Copyright © March 1989 by Newton Hightower.

Deane Juhan from his *Job's Body: A Handbook for Bodywork.* Station Hill Press. Copyright © 1987 by Deane Juhan.

Alexander and Leslie Lowen from their *The Way to Vibrant Health: A Manual of Bioenergetic Exercises.* Harper & Row. Copyright © 1977 by Alexander and Leslie Lowen.

Mayfield Publishing Company from *Won't You Join in The Dance?* by Trudi Schoop. Copyright © 1974 by Mayfield Publishing Co.

Plenum Publishing Co. from *The Exercise Prescription For Depression and Anxiety* by Keith W. Jöhnsgard. Copyright © 1989 by Plenum Publishing Co.

Random House from *Women Who Run With The Wolves* by Clarissa Pinkola Estés. Ballantine Books. Copyright © 1992 by Clarissa Pinkola Estés.

Lynn Redgrave from her play *Shakespeare For My Father* (to be published). Copyright © 1994 by Lynn Redgrave.

Geneen Roth from her *Breaking Free From Compulsive Eating.* North American Library. Copyright © 1986 by Geneen Roth.

Edward W.L. Smith from his The Body In Psychotherapy. McFarland & Company, Inc. Publishers, Jefferson, NC 28640. Copyright © 1985 by Edward W.L. Smith.

Index

A

abuse
  and changes in breathing 103
  and global autobiographical memory impairment 67–68
  and importance of bodywork 83–84
  effects on biological development 32
  surviving by dissociation 73–74
Ackerman, Diane 69, 88, 245
action stage 49
addictions 34–35
  anger 229
  blocking natural emotional expressions 80
  five stages for changing behavior 48–50
  learning to do nothing 175–78
  sex 241
Aikido 89, 91
Alexander Technique 89
alexithymia 61
aliveness
  maintaining 275–79
amnesia 75
Angelou, Maya 71–72
anger
  and rage 226, 234
  applying hydraulic theory 228
  as an addiction 229
  fear of 226, 228, 235

  handling rage with awareness 227–28
  managing 225–38
  women holding in 227
anger management exercises
  Cooling the fire with water 233–34
  for ragers 229–33
  Get off my back 235–36
  No! No! No! 237–38
  Turn off the road to anger 231–33
animal energy 132
anxiety
  addressing through bodywork 87
  and breathing difficulty 108
  chemical treatment of 81
  effect of exercise on 123
appreciation exercises
  Different bodies 195–96
  Learning to appreciate 193–95
asthma 33, 101, 108
Aston-Patterning 89

B

Benson, Herbert 258
bioenergetics 89, 102
Blemish game 197–98
blood pressure
  effects of venting anger 226–27
body
  angst about body image 188
  appreciating 183–84
  as teacher 27–28
  awareness of 61

About the Author

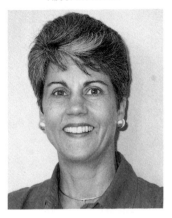

Rita Justice, Ph.D., is a clinical psychologist who has been in private practice in Houston for twenty-two years. With her husband, psychologist Dr. Blair Justice, she co-authored two pioneering books on child abuse and incest (*The Abusing Family*, Human Sciences Press, 1976, and a revised edition in 1990, Plenum; *The Broken Taboo: Sex in the Family*, Human Sciences Press, 1979). She is on the adjunct faculty in pediatrics at Baylor College of Medicine and The Union Institute. Dr. Justice has lectured and taught extensively in this country and internationally. From the beginning of her clinical practice, she has kept the body as well as the mind and emotions an important focus in her psychotherapeutic work. When not practicing psychology, writing, conducting workshops, and lecturing, Dr. Justice and her husband enjoy mountain climbing, travel, classical music, and playing with Tashi, their Tibetan terrier.

Order Form

I want _____ copies of *ALIVE AND WELL* at $16.00 each plus $4.50 shipping per book. (Texas residents please include 8 1/4% state sales tax.)Canadian orders must be accompanied by a postal money order in U.S. funds. Allow 30 days for delivery.

Name _____

Phone _____

Address _____

City/State/Zip _____

Credit Card ❏ Mastercard ❏ Visa

Card # _____

Expires _____

Name on card (Print)_____

Signature _____

Check or money order enclosed ❏

Total order amount $

Please make your check payable to:

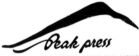

Peak press

2402 Westgate Drive, Suite 200
Houston, Texas 77019

CHECK YOUR BOOKSTORE OR CALL YOUR ORDER TO:
(713) 528-6571 FAX (713) 5296577